ON NURSING:
A LITERARY CELEBRATION

ON NURSING:
A LITERARY CELEBRATION
An Anthology

Editors and Authors
Margretta Madden Styles
Patricia Moccia

Consulting Editor
Nancy Evans

National League for Nursing • New York
Pub. No. 14-2512

CREDITS

Achterberg, J. Excerpts from WOMAN AS HEALER by Jeanne Achterberg. Copyright © 1990 by Jeanne Achterberg. Reprinted by arrangement with Shambhala Publications, 300 Massachusetts Avenue, Boston MA 02115.

Alexander, M. W. From the book *I Dream a World: Portraits of Black Women Who Changed America,* copyright © 1989, Brian Lanker. Reprinted by permission of Stewart, Tabori & Chang, Publishers, New York.

Allende, I. "Interminable life." Reprinted with the permission of Atheneum Publishers, an imprint of Macmillan Publishing Company from THE STORIES OF EVA LUNA by Isabel Allende, translated from the Spanish by Margaret Sayers Peden. Copyright © 1991 by Isabel Allende. English translation copyright © 1991 by Macmillan Publishing Company.

(Credits continued on page 341.)

ISBN 0-88737-574-X

The views expressed in this publication represent the views of the authors and do not necessarily reflect the official views of the National League for Nursing.

Printed in the United States of America

CONTENTS

Publisher's Foreword

> . . . to share and spread also those words that are
> meaningful to us.

> Audre Lorde, *Sister Outsider,* 1984

Audre Lorde died this year. No, she was not a member of the National League for Nursing, had not ever presented at one of our conferences, and probably had not even been aware of the existence of the League, much less that 1993 marks our centennial. Although there is some record that she had at one time considered becoming a practical nurse, she is not mentioned in this foreword for her direct connection with nursing or the League.

Audre Lorde was a self-proclaimed "warrior"; who fought, through her passionate writings and activist's life, against the "tyrannies of silence," which would separate us, one from the other and each from our communities and, in so doing, distort the historical forces of freedom. She wrote as a strong African American woman, a clear feminist, and a lesbian mother, with word patterns that exposed the myths of our society to all who, by chance or deliberate choice, read her works. Her power, like Antigone's, was from her clear vision of where true loyalties lie, a vision sharpened from living outside America's mythical norm that we are all "white, thin, male, young, heterosexual, Christian, and financially secure." Her life's work, once read, places Lorde within our consciousness forever, informing our own struggles against the "tyrannies" she contested and sustaining, nourishing, and leading us to choices of liberation.

I speak of Audre Lorde in this foreword because her life project parallels the life project of those who choose to create their space in the world as nurses. Throughout our history, now as then, the National League for Nursing has been the vehicle for the expression of strong individuals who chose to create their own community, where caring and courage and passionate activism were valued and wherein they were sustained, nourished, and lead by these words. This book is but the latest expression of the commitment of the National League for Nursing to this community.

But this book is more because the National League for Nursing of today and tomorrow must be more. Throughout the past hundred years until today, not all of those within our community have benefited from its riches; nor have all had the same opportunity to care for their communities, to lead their profession, to live their lives as nurses as fully as their talents would enable them. Instead, many have been suffered to fight for their place among us with the weight of racism sapping precious energies; they have looked to their sisters, too, and seen the face of oppression. And we have too long been silent.

Audre Lorde's words begin this Publisher's Foreword in a tribute to her life's work which was "an attempt to break that silence and bridge some of the differences between us." The National League for Nursing proudly publishes this book as the symbol of its direction at the beginning of our second century, in recognition of "our responsibility to seek those words out, to read them and to share them and examine them in pertinence to our lives"—those words that will transform the silence as Lorde wrote, "into language and action"; words, such as those that follow, that will transform the silence into health and healing.

Patricia Moccia

New York
June 1993

ACKNOWLEDGMENTS

We have never before prepared an anthology nor attempted a project of such sweeping scope in time, geography, and subject. We have learned much in the process, principally that such an undertaking is a team effort.

For example, we have discovered that the services of a consulting editor are indispensable. In this case, Nancy Evans, well-known to nurses as an editor and writer for health care publications, was invaluable in locating and circulating the pieces of literature for our consideration and selection. Beyond this vital contribution, she cheered us on, managed much of the complicated process, and guided us through the tough choices we had to make from the mounds of published and unpublished literature reviewed. We might mention, by the way, that we had not expected nominators to recommend such a large assortment of unpublished writing. The fact that we received many such offerings and selected a small number for inclusion suggests that there are not enough publishing outlets for "nursing humanities" literature or that nurses are not accustomed to submitting material to such sources.

Patricia Struckman served as editorial associate and "perfecter" of what must have been one of the world's most complex manuscripts. The documentation and the formatting are Herculean tasks in preparing a publication of this nature. Pat also handled correspondence with the global community of nurses invited to recommend their favorite literature, as well as correspondence with authors and publishers to secure the permissions to use copyrighted material.

Family and friends were pressed into service, according to their special talents. Doug Styles did whatever needed to be done, from critiquing early drafts to keeping the mail circulating throughout the team. Meg Styles-Rogers, a university student with an interest in a nursing career, evaluated candidate literature from the student perspective. Joseph Madden, a retired English professor, reviewed each chapter with a curious and critical eye. Hazel Georgetti, Kelly Birch, and Suzanne Struckman assisted in the voluminous typing when deadlines were upon us.

Above all, we are indebted to the hundreds of nurses from the USA and around the world who answered our call to identify for us the literature most beautiful and most meaningful to them. We would like them to recognize *On Nursing: A Literary Celebration* as their collective masterpiece.

And, we hope, not immodestly, that we acknowledge one another for sharing a vision and a commitment. In effect, we held up the canvas and invited the world of nursing to portray itself in magnificent literary splendor.

MARGRETTA MADDEN STYLES
PATRICIA MOCCIA

ABOUT THE AUTHORS

Margretta Madden Styles, EdD, RN, FAAN, is former dean and professor emeritus, School of Nursing, University of California, San Francisco. She is past president, American Nurses Association and current member, board of directors, International Council of Nurses. She holds honorary membership in the Institute of Medicine, National Academy of Sciences. She is an Honorary Fellow, Royal College of Nursing, United Kingdom, and holds honorary doctoral degrees from Valpariso University, Indiana, and the University of Athens, Greece.

Patricia Moccia, PhD, RN, FAAN, is the chief operating officer and executive vice president of the National League for Nursing. She is a renowned educator, public speaker, author, and a leading force in curriculum revolution for nursing schools across the nation. Her most recent post is as adjunct professor at the Union for Experimenting Colleges and Universities. Dr. Moccia is known for her work over the past 25 years as a feminist and political activist on all the major social, health, and economic issues of our time.

Nancy Evans, BS, has been immersed in publishing for nurses and other health professionals for more than three decades. She has been associated with The Mosby Company, Addison-Wesley, and Appleton and Lange, sponsoring many award-winning, best-selling nursing books and teaching seminars and workshops on writing and publishing. Now an independent writer, editor, and publishing consultant, she lives in San Francisco. She is an honorary member of Sigma Theta Tau.

I

INTRODUCTION

❦

THE IMPORTANCE OF A LITERATURE ON NURSING

A profession devoted to human welfare and social betterment must cultivate, savor, and proclaim the literature that forms and expresses its character. It is timely and necessary, especially as nursing struggles for its identity within a technology-dominated, science-driven, crisis-oriented environment, that the profession tend to its humanities, that nursing define the body of literature that defines its culture.

In his book, *In the Country of Hearts,* John Stone describes the many purposes that literature can serve for health professionals. Translating his words to the world of nursing, we are told:

- A powerful resonance must occur between nursing and literature.

- Nurses and writers draw from the same sources: from the human encounter, from people and their indelible stories, and from the skillful use of the senses.

- Literature has a laboratory function, in that a person's life can be thought of as a series of stories, coalescing over time to form the most idiosyncratic novel ever written.

1

- Literature can provide for students . . . catharsis, personal insights, and support.
- Literature is not extracurricular; it is hard data, not soft.
- Literature provides opportunity for reflection.
- The writing of literature is therapeutic in and of itself.

(Adapted from Stone, 1990, pp. 67–71)

On Nursing: A Literary Celebration introduces a body of literature to serve as laboratory, provocateur, catharsis, and support for nurses. This anthology has been compiled thoughtfully and lovingly for students seeking their identity and place in the professional community; for nurses probing deeper into their calling or facing professional dilemmas; for scholars wishing to understand a profession searching for its métier in a changing and sometimes chaotic world; and for the millions who are touched by nursing every day.

It is hoped that *On Nursing* will spark a nursing and literature movement, and that nursing schools will take up the call to educate and socialize undergraduate and graduate students by infusing literature throughout the curriculum and/or offering specific "nursing literature or humanities" courses or units. Reading and writing literature puts a human face on the technical biopsychosocial content and deepens the meaning of nursing. Learning through literature leads to a more broadly educated nurse, whose life will be enriched, whose practice will be enhanced, and whose standing within the ranks of professionals will be elevated.

And it is hoped that nurses will take up their pens (or personal computers) and write their own stories, journals, essays, poems. Thus, *On Nursing* will always be unfinished, as it is incomplete. It is a core around which layers of literature will accumulate piece by piece as nurses and nursing continue to define their destiny.

ON NURSING AND YOU

On Nursing draws on all literary forms—poems, biographies, essays, books, articles, editorials, stories—spanning centuries, cultures, and nations. These pieces of literature were gathered by combing the libraries and by soliciting suggestions from more than 1,000 nurses in the United States and around the world. The names of the respondents are listed in Appendix A, with the grateful acknowledgment of the editors. From the substantial volume of published and unpublished literature thus identified, selections were made, essentially based on three components: the quality of expression, the nature of the message, and the degree of balance among subjects. The title emerged from our finding that there is truly much to celebrate about and within the literature that is meaningful to nurses.

Inasmuch as the literature has no inherent morphology, such a book can only be organized arbitrarily. Therefore, we have selected a scheme that seemed to flow from the content. You are invited to read from front to back or to roam randomly through the pages or to choose purposefully from the table of contents and index. Educators might use the entire volume as the centerpiece for an introductory course on nursing and literature, or selections could be used throughout the nursing curriculum to humanize and extend learning. A chapter on writing has been added to challenge readers to augment the nursing literature as well as to partake of it.

We have interwoven and punctuated the pieces with a running narrative. We hope that you, too, will "speak" to the literature and that you will be drawn into conversation with the writers of these selections. To give countenance and context to the dialogue, a brief profile of the author appears when the writer's work is first introduced.

We invite you to hold and caress *On Nursing,* inhale its essence, reach into its pages, read its words, listen to its voice, mine its meanings, add to its significance, and forge our bond to nursing and to the needy world that nursing touches so eloquently. The most we could hope for, as you submerge yourself in this literature, is expressed in Wallace Stevens' poem (1965), *The House Was Quiet and the World Was Calm:* "and the reader became the book." May you become the book.

II

ON LITERATURE AND NURSING

What is literature? How does it stand out from other writing? Literature, experts explain, is writing characterized by its excellence in form or expression or by its ideas of permanent or universal interest. We would add that literature, as contrasted with formal (and sometimes formidable) textbooks or technical reports, invites the reader into wide-ranging discourse, reaching for depths of understanding or feeling. From a scientific text, for example, we might come to know findings to date about the physiology of senescence. From literature, we can know the experience of aging and perceptions about the aged.

Literature provides a vital connection between the professional and the lay person, because it is interesting and understandable to both. Literature divides us not by professions or disciplines, but by the degree of development of our intellect, sensitivity, and appreciation.

Literature is enduring, though not ageless. It may well reflect and be instructive of the time in which it was written. However, the beauty, cogency, and poignancy of its content are lasting.

Literature is an anthropological dig; within it are embedded layers of ancient and modern cultural nuances and values to be discovered, examined, and remembered.

Being a member of the *literati,* the broadly educated, the well-read, is not something to be shunned or denied. It is not even a choice to be made. Honing our intellect and understanding through delving into literature, as we have defined it above, enriches our practice as professionals—indeed, marks us as professionals.

This chapter could be compared to a play within a play; it is composed of literature about literature and its role in humanizing professions.

*   *   *

WHAT IS A PROFESSION?

EARLE P. SCARLETT (1896–1982). Canadian physician, writer, and medical historian. An authority on John Keats and Sir Arthur Conan Doyle, Dr. Scarlett was long fascinated by the interplay between medicine and the arts.

The truth of the matter is that any profession worthy of the name must forever be strengthening and re-creating its traditions. A profession is a sensitive organic growing thing, not a static order. And it is particularly important that we should remember this at the present time. The two great wars have disinherited and confused a multitude of sensitive minds, with the result that they have tended to lose their sense of the past and of the future. They are acquiring an experience of life not easily related to the great achievements of time past and to the ancestral wisdom of man. In consequence, they are without roots.

Man is a time-binding animal and lives in three dimensions of time as well as of space. To maintain this point of vantage, we must constantly recover and build perspective. This neglected, a condition of things results in which perspective is lost and man comes to exist for the immediate present only. When this happens, it can have disastrous effects in a profession, reducing it to a time-serving trade, and producing in the individual a sense of futility and disillusion. (p. 119)

Scarlett describes seven pillars of a profession, among them

The fourth: a knowledge of literature and the arts. This acts as a catalyst; here are to be found the world of values and the repository of what has been said and done by the best minds. Such knowledge provides a philosophy of excellence, and insight that comes from sensitiveness. It is well to remember, looking back no further than the years of this century, that the barbarians do not destroy science and technology. They destroy the vessels of liberal culture—the roots of the past—libraries, the press, religion, music, art, the belief in the essential dignity of man. (p. 120)

In the following plaintive editorial, this author recounts how nursing leaders have, over the decades, made an appeal for recognition of the relationship between nursing and the humanities, that is, the cultural branches of learning, as distinguished from the sciences.

THE SPIRIT OF NURSING

M. PATRICIA DONAHUE, a contemporary nurse historian, is an associate professor at the University of Iowa College of Nursing, and editor of Nursing: The Finest Art *(1985), an illustrated history of nursing.*

The caring component of nursing encompasses much more than a combination of the scientific and the technical. It encompasses and mandates a balance of "the head, the heart, and the hands" or "the science, the skill, and the spirit." We have forged ahead in the areas of science and technology, but there is fear among us that this spirit becomes dimmer and dimmer with the passage of time. And yet, according to Stewart[1] . . . that spirit was essential to the development of the nursing art.

The real essence of nursing, as of any fine art, lies not in the mechanical details of execution, nor yet in the dexterity of the performer, but in the creative imagination, the sensitive spirit, and the intelligent understanding lying back of these techniques and skills. Without these, nursing may become a highly skilled trade, but it cannot be a profession or a fine art. All the rituals and ceremonials which our modern worship of efficiency may devise, and all our elaborate scientific equipment will not save us if the intellectual and spiritual elements in our art are subordinated to the mechanical, and if the means come to be regarded as more important than ends.

Nursing has its roots in the humanities, which address the wholeness of the persons for whom we care. Nursing has been sanctioned by society; nursing care satisfies a real human need. Nursing mandates the interaction with people at the most intimate level during the most crucial and critical times in their lives. And yet, the liberal arts in our educational programs continue to diminish to accommodate the scientific knowledge necessary to practice nursing. We seem to have forgotten the struggle of our early leaders to incorporate the liberal arts, the humanities within the mainstream of nursing. They, too, were concerned that the spirit of our work be kept alive. Isabel M. Stewart, in particular, feared for the loss of the humanitarian aspects that have long been a vital force in nursing. Recognizing that a definite decline in the study of the area was occurring, she commented in a letter to Lillian A. Hudson (c. 1940–1947):

I feel very strongly these days that we are failing to develop the social and humanistic side of nursing . . . the spirit of nursing as we used to call it . . . and all that goes to the balancing of the scientific and technical aspects . . . it would mean a restudy of that whole area dealing with the philosophy and history of nursing and the social sciences, and the strengthening of our cultural roots, both in nursing schools (basic) and in the preparation of graduate nurses for developing this phase of nursing.

Perhaps it is finally time to remind ourselves that we are where we are because of the vision of persons in our heritage and to ask ourselves whether that vision has been sustained. Or whether the spirit or art of caring is slowly disappearing at a time within our society when the focus on humanness should be paramount. Is something vital to nursing's social mission missing?

The "Spirit of Nursing" is uniquely and poignantly represented in a place that might seem somewhat unusual. This Nurses Memorial framed by stately trees majestically stands on a grassy knoll in Arlington National Cemetery in Virginia. Rising 8 feet 6 inches above the ground, the Memorial overlooks the graves of nurses from the Spanish-American War through Vietnam who are buried on the hillside below, thus commemorating the devoted service to our country by Army, Navy, and Air Force nurses. The words spoken at the dedication of this monument in 1938 serve to remind nurses of the importance of this facet of nursing:[2] "Their tenderness and compassion, their competence, courage and human qualities . . . the spirit of nursing of the past, of today, and of the years to come." (p. 149)

HUMANISTIC NURSING

JOSEPHINE PATERSON and LORETTA ZDERAD are nurse researchers with respective interests in public health and psychiatric nursing. Their theory of nursing evolved from a course on humanistic nursing taught in 1972 at the Veterans Administration Hospital in Northport, NY.

When arts and humanities are included in nursing education programs, it is for their humanizing effects. Traditionally they have been recognized as having a civilizing influence. So in nursing they are seen as supporting the elements of humanness and humanitarianism. Furthermore, they are a necessary antidote for the depersonalization that accompanies scientific technology and mechanization . . . . They stimulate imaginative creativity. They broaden a person's perspective of the human situation, of man in his world. For instance, depictions of suffering man or of other aspects of the human condition that are found in poetry, drama, or literature are far more descriptive and much closer to reality than those given in typical textbooks.

Currently nursing practice reflects the educational preparation of nurses that is weighted heavily with scientific courses and the methodology of positivistic science. Arts and humanities are a necessary complement. Science aims at universals and the discovery of general laws; art reveals the uniqueness of the individual. While science strives for quantification, art is more concerned with quality. Strict conformance to methodology and replicability are prized in scientific studies, whereas freedom and uniqueness of style reign in art. Science, forever updating itself, opens the nurse's eyes to constant change and innovation; the classics promote a sense of the unchanging and lasting in man's world. Science may provide the nurse with knowledge on which to base her decision, but it remains for the arts and humanities to direct the nurse toward examination of value underlying her practice.[3] (p. 87)

> As is illustrated in two fine selections below, nurses and physicians alike have extolled the centrality of the arts, and in particular, poetry, in their clinical practice.

THE ART OF THE MATTER

VENETA MASSON is a nurse and the director of Community Medical Care, a family medical and nursing practice in Washington, DC. This editorial appeared in Nursing Outlook *in 1991.*

It was the Sixties and I was a student of everything. I had an Associate Degree in nursing and a year of hospital experience under my belt. I had moved to the California Bay Area and enrolled first at University of California, Berkeley, then at the Medical Center campus in San Francisco. I was drenched in new knowledge. I felt shiny and new and very wise. I was 21.

Revelations in Verse

There was a paperback book of poetry I used to carry around with me. In it, I found a short poem by William Stafford called "Strokes." It began like this:

> The left side of her world is gone—
> the rest sustained by memory

and a realization: There are still the
children.[4]

Now, I had nursed stroke patients. Their care held no mysteries
for me—until I read the poem. The more I read it, the more I became convinced that only if I really, truly understood what that
poem was saying, could I nurse a stroke patient. This certainty
grew inside me until I could scarcely contain it.

That semester I was taking Psych 110 with Louis Schaw, an *enfant
terrible* who used to play the class with the same diabolical skill
that Paganini is said to have played the violin. In discussion, he
would lure you down a path you'd never taken before, through
dense thickets, across vast plains, up high mountains, then, without warning, just as you were about to reach the summit, he'd
turn on you and challenge your right to be there. I seldom spoke
in class. But one afternoon, when the topic had turned to what
nursing is, my hand shot up, my mouth opened, and I heard myself telling about the poem and what it had taught me about nursing. Dr. Schaw allowed the briefest of silences after I had finished,
then fixed me in his sights. "Aren't you being rather naive?" he
asked. And he went on to describe the command of technology
and the skills one needs to make the diagnosis of CVA, stabilize
the patient's vital signs, restore function, and prevent complications and further losses. An admirable display of medical expertise for a professor of psychology!

I was struck dumb. What he said was true. But was it the whole
truth? Instead of letting go, I only held on tighter to my revelation.
I knew what I knew. But it would be my secret.

In the years that followed, I did not run across any other poems
or works of art that had the same impact on me. I remember
reading Kafka's "Metamorphosis" in a graduate nursing course at
the University of Washington, but I had trouble relating it to the
care of patients who, in my experience, rarely turned into cock-
roaches. After graduate school, I drifted away from hands-on
nursing. I would see occasional references in the literature to a
novel or short story of use in helping students acquire empathy

with patients. None of these works were actually written by nurses. I didn't find that remarkable. Then.

By 1980, I was back again, a clinician involved in hospice care, home care, and primary health care. I found myself brooding about patients who troubled or perplexed me. There was one in particular, an elderly woman, poor, bedbound, living alone in a rundown house that strangers used to deal and shoot drugs. More than one health professional counseled me to withdraw my services and "precipitate a crisis" so that the city could step in and force her into a nursing home "where she belonged." And yet, there was something about this woman that was compelling: she had expectations. She owned her own home and owned her grave plot and planned to go from one to the other when the Lord called her. Not before. One evening after dinner, utterly frustrated, I pulled out my journal and began to write:

> Just
> who do you think you are, Maggie
> Jones, following me home from work,
> insinuating yourself into my evening,
> shading my thoughts?

Over time, Maggie turned into a long narrative poem.[5] And as she did, I began to understand her, and myself when I was with her. I believe that, as a result, I was able to nurse her really, truly.

Sold Out to Technology

After Maggie, other patients of mine, past and present, started turning into poems. It could happen at any time, without warning, like the day Aretha Robbins, in the depths of depression, told me as we sat at her dining room table:

> There are three ways to do it—
> (Do what? do what?)
> jump out the window
> poison or . . . you know . . .
> (What do I know?)

> This! she said
> and flicked one scarred wrist
> with a whisk
> of the other hand.

It's art—my own poetry for the most part—that enables me to nurse Carol with AIDS, Maria with chronic pelvic pain, and Curtis who, at eight, has never tasted grapes, or love. It's art that sustains me in a profession that many of my colleagues contemplate leaving. It's art that expresses what drew me to nursing in the first place and connects me with every other nurse. I submit that the heart of nursing is the art of nursing, and to quote Wordsworth, "we have given our hearts away." We've sold out to technology, like everyone else.

Art Holds the Power to Unite Nurses

We are two million strong—and that doesn't count practical nurses and nursing assistants who also nurse. We work in every nook and cranny of the health care system. We have researchers, educators, managers, clinical specialists. We have politicians, pundits, and entrepreneurs. What we need now are a few poets, playwrights, visual artists—maybe a musician or two. To nurse—really, truly—is art, and our art holds the power we need to unite us, keep us going, move us forward. It's time, high time, to unleash it. (p. 187)

THE POETRY OF MEDICINE

> *JULIE FISHBEIN, a physician and writer who won the First Annual William Carlos Williams Poetry Competition for Medical Students in 1983, published this essay in the* Journal of the American Medical Association *in 1990.*

In 1985 I went to graduate school to become a writer. It was a fascinating time for me, surrounded by famous poets, and everyone involved in the act of making art. In fact, everyone was writing about the process of art, writing poetry about writing poetry. But I soon felt something was missing in the poems, something vital and vibrant, which I couldn't quite pinpoint.

Until I returned to medicine, and there it was in every room. I want to take you there, to one particular 10 × 12-foot room on the pediatric ward, a spacious room for a short stay. My friend Sarah lives there. Sarah is 3 years old. She has aplastic anemia. You can spot her any day in her red plastic high-heeled slippers, costume jewelry, and underwear, as she comes clickety-clack down the hall. Sarah can't read, but we often find her sitting at the nurses' station, thumbing through her own hospital chart, considering each page carefully. If you need to borrow the chart, you must ask her permission and be prepared to come back later. She is a powerful child.

And yet I have seen her meek and too breathless to speak, with a circle of relatives joined in prayer around her bed. These are the vicissitudes of her illness.

There is no use putting on airs with her. She will call your bluff. The first time I met her it was 2 in the morning, and the nurse had called to tell me Sarah had a fever. I ambled sleepily to her room, examined her, and explained matter-of-factly that I needed to draw some blood. As I reached into my pockets for the things I needed, Sarah peered up at me from her tangle of IVs like a little spider in her web and asked, just as matter-of-factly, if I was *sure* I knew what I was doing.

I had to stop and think. She knew full well the physician's fallibility, and I never forgot that confrontation. The next day she stopped on her go-cart to tell me I'd done a good job. Thank you, Sarah.

Sarah's mother has just had twins. She was hoping one of them would be a match for a bone marrow transplant, which is Sarah's only chance for a cure. But neither is. So now the room has three little girls, and Sarah's mom jokes about buying a farm to put all the kids on, all the kids she may have to find for a match for Sarah. Sarah's dad has gotten a job in the hospital's maintenance department. They will never afford a farm, but their hospital room is one of the richest places on Earth. I go there often, and it nourishes me.

There is a great deal of voyeurism in medicine, and I have come to enjoy it, to be unembarrassed by it.

You walk into a room with a set of questions in your mind; you want to answer the riddle of the illness, to make a diagnosis. But each time you are surprised. You find the answers enveloped in a scene, a family under stress in a little room whose boundaries compress and confine them like the lines of a poem.

As they struggle to answer your questions, as they probe for your opinions and, at the same time, judge you, as they work together (or against one another), joke and pray and curse and cry their way through a troubling time, they are making a poem of their lives. They are creating scenes that brand themselves into your memory. They are offering you what William Carlos Williams called "an intimation of what is going on in the world," or the lesson that Kierkegaard wanted so much to learn: "how to live a life."

The essence of all poetry is in that room. In the naked patient standing before you, you see yourself and your own mortality. It is a confrontation. The atmosphere is charged, and every gesture belies greater things moving beneath the surface.

So what am I trying to tell you about medicine and poetry? Just, I suppose, that they are inextricably linked, that I have found more poetry here than in all the ivory towers. Each room I enter is a living poem, struggling to create itself. I am a witness to my patients, they are my teachers, and to learn from them is the greatest privilege I know. (p. 2999)

Notes

1. Stewart, I. M. (1929). The science and art of nursing (editorial). *Nursing Education Bulletin, 2,* 1.
2. Nurses' monument unveiled in Arlington (1939). *American Journal of Nursing, 39,* 90.

3. Paterson, J. G., & Zderad, L. T. (1988). *Humanistic nursing* (p. 87). New York: National League for Nursing.
4. Hall, D. (1962). *Contemporary American Poetry.* Baltimore, MD: Penguin Books.
5. Masson, V. (1987, March). Maggie Jones. *Journal of Christian Nursing,* 22–24.

III

ON WOMEN AND WORK

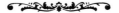

*E*very man's work, whether it be literature or music or pictures or architecture or anything else, is always a portrait of himself.

Samuel Butler, *The Way of All Flesh,* 1903

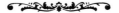

Working and women's work are two concepts central to nursing.

The perceived significance of their field of work and their place within it is a defining aspect of all persons, as Butler has proclaimed above. Literature on work, therefore, helps explore and establish one's self-concept as a worker.

What is written about women and their work holds at least two inextricable meanings for nurses. The majority of nurses around the world are women, although the size of that majority varies from country to country. The nature of nursing and the role and status of nurses are tied to the historic and universal view of nursing as women's work—nurturing in character, ubiquitous and amorphous in scope, often secondary in standing. Thus, the literature on women and work pertains equally to men and women in nursing and how they discern their context, their craft, their challenges, and their inherent assets and liabilities in meeting those challenges.

Women, in revealing the inseparability of their nature and their work, have written eloquently, but often in a pensive, tentative mode. In rich and poor nation alike, from generation to generation, culture by culture, cutting across occupational settings and hierarchies, there is a sameness of theme and affect, with variations in intensity and subtlety.

*   *   *

Facts for Life, a UNICEF/WHO/UNESCO publication written to empower families to use today's knowledge to protect children, has summed up the situation in the developing world.

WOMEN'S WORK

Putting today's essential health knowledge into practice will be seen by many as "women's work."

But women already have work.

They already grow most of the developing world's food, market most of its crops, fetch most of its water, collect most of its fuel, feed most of its animals, weed most of its fields.

And when their work outside the home is done, they light the third world's fires, cook its meals, clean its compounds, wash its clothes, shop for its needs, and look after its old and its ill.

And they bear and care for its children.

The multiple burdens of womanhood are too much.

And the greatest communications challenge of all is the challenge of communicating the idea that the time has come, in all countries, for men to share more fully in that most difficult and important of all tasks—protecting the lives and the health and the growth of their children.

Facts for Life is therefore addressed not only to women but to men.

WOMAN AS HEALER

JEANNE ACHTERBERG, author of Imagery in Healing, *is professor of psychology at the Institute of Transpersonal Psychology, and has served as associate professor and director of research in rehabilitation at the University of Texas Southwestern Medical School in Dallas. This selection is taken from her 1990 work,* Woman as Healer.

The Thread of Consciousness of Woman as Healer

A thread of consciousness weaves through the centuries, connecting one era of women healers to the next. It relates to the feminine myth—the behaviors, abilities, and belief systems traditionally associated with women. Whether the myth originates in culture or ·biology is debatable and somewhat irrelevant—it simply is. In terms of healing, the feminine myth relates to such attributes as intuition, nurturance, and compassion. When expressed in professional practice, it supports the virtues of nature as healing resources, and the curative aspects of caring.

Women demonstrate the feminine myth in their choice of healing techniques and medicaments. They tend to be empiricists, observing at the bedside what soothes and heals and what does not. Their choice of profession is based on these observations; they gravitate to fields emphasizing prevention and the gentler botanics (rather than aggressive procedures), and to those serving the needs of other women and their children. The feminine myth supports the use of ritual at life's passages to acknowledge human bonds and the infinite connection of life.

Now and again, the feminine healing myth—the consciousness of woman as healer—moves brilliantly ungirded into the world, touching and changing and healing the space of humanity in ever-widening circles. Then, trapped by twisted logic and primal fears, by power's perverse seduction of human beings, it retreats. . . .

During the past few years, the expression of the feminine myth in healing has become more resolute and has taken on new dimensions. Women of a special caliber—the vast majority well-trained professionals—are appearing in great numbers.

They can be found working in hospital emergency rooms, and well-baby clinics, and hospices. They staff shelters for battered women and victims of rape. They minister to congregations and teach students. They are everywhere—in the creative arts, in the social sciences, in allied health professions. They heal with their hands and their words and their deep conviction that they have a knowledge or talent that will help others in some way.

Their work is likely to reflect a broad sense of healing that aspires to wholeness or harmony within the self, the family, and the global community. They see body, mind, and spirit as the inseparable nature of humankind; they believe that any healing ministrations have an impact on each element of this triune nature. They regard sickness as a potential catalyst for both emotional and spiritual growth, among other things. These healers have chosen to accompany, help, lead, teach, and care for others who seek wholeness.

These women view healing not as something one does to another, but as a process that takes place through the healer/healee relationship. Healing relates not so much to techniques as to philosophic and spiritual foundations. The bond that is established between the healer of this genre and the healee is life-giving and life-enriching for both. The relationship, itself, is held in reverence, with the awareness that it is made of trust, love, and hope. They aver that they are, indeed, working in sacred space.

The emergence of women whose consciousness blends with the ancient themes of healing is the single most promising event in health care, for the lack of a feminine point of view is the most abject omission in American institutions and at the heart of the problems in American medicine. The manifestation of feminine values in medicine is critical for the health of the planet.

The women healers who share the thread of consciousness have taken a major leap forward from the past: they know that the feminine myth must influence, but not replace, advanced technology and sound, scientific strategies for helping and healing at all levels—physical, mental, and spiritual. The invisible spaces are seen as sacred, but so is good medicine, good counseling, good science, or whatever is being used to facilitate wellness. To return exclusively to the feminine myth in healing is to return to the Dark Ages. It is to be expected, then, that women healers are being joined in their mission by compassionate, nurturing, intuitive men who desire balance in their lives and in their professions. (pp. 3–5)

> Across the generations, women have whispered to one another, and occasionally shouted, to pass along the lessons of their lives and work.

TAPESTRIES OF LIFE

BETTINA APTHEKER, a transplanted New Yorker living in Northern California, is a professor of women's studies at the University of California, Santa Cruz. In addition to Tapestries of Life *(1989), she is the author of* Women's Legacy: Essays on Race, Sex, and Class in American History.

Women's everyday lives are often fragmented and dispersed, caught up short between a job, dinner, and the laundry. They are often episodic. That is, they are often determined by events outside of women's control, such as the opening or closing of a factory in which most of them and/or their husbands are employed. Likewise, women are frequently required to move from city to city or country to country, uprooting family and community, because their husbands' corporate, professional, or military assignments are relocated. Women are continually interrupted. Projects, especially their own, are put aside to be completed on another day or in another year. In the course of a day, a week, women carry the threads of many tasks in their hands at the same time. Poet Deena Metzger once wrote: **"Each day is a tapestry, threads of broccoli, promotion, couches, children, politics, shopping, building, planting, thinking interweave in intimate connection with insistent cycles of birth, existence, and death."**[1] Some of these things also happen to men, but not all of them, and they don't happen in the same ways because most men . . . are not ultimately responsible for maintaining personal relationships and networks. They are not primarily responsible for emotional work. They are not primarily responsible for the children, the elders, the relatives, the holidays, the cooking, the cleaning, the shopping, the mending, the laundry. Their position as men, even as working-class men and men of color, gives them access to more resources and status relative to the women and families of their communities because the society institutionalizes a system of male domination.

By the dailiness of women's lives I mean the patterns women create and the meanings women invent each day and over time as a result of their labors and in the context of their subordinated status to men. The point is not to describe every aspect of daily life or to represent a schedule of priorities in which some activities are more important or accorded more status than others. The point is to suggest a way of knowing from the meanings women give to their labors. The search for dailiness is a method of work that allows us to take the patterns women create and the meanings women invent and learn from them. If we map what we learn, connecting one meaning or invention to another, we begin to lay out a different way of seeing reality. This way of seeing is what I refer to as women's standpoint.[2] And this standpoint pivots, of course, depending upon the class, cultural, or racial locations of its subjects, and upon their age, sexual preference, physical abilities, the nature of their work and personal relationships. What is proposed is a mapping of that which has been traditionally erased or hidden.

To find a starting point for this map we may turn back to our mothers. . . . In this turning we see that many of our mothers sacrificed, worked hard, nurtured, did the best they could to "make do," to improve the quality of our daily lives. We also know that some of our mothers died before we were grown. We see that others of our mothers were alcoholic, abusive, emotionally distant. We see that some of our mothers abandoned us as children. We see that some of our mothers were materially privileged but spiritually impoverished. From all of these stories we learn about the reality of women's lives, about the suffering, the failure, the struggle to nurture well. We learn about how other women took care of children who were not their own—grandmothers and aunts, friends and older sisters—women who just took over the child care and did the best they could to raise us. In the conflict between mothers and daughters we learn about the ways in which women are divided from each other, about how we are taught to compete with each other. All of this speaks to women's social condition, to women's social reality enforced by class, by race, by the prescription of gendered roles, inscribed in the dailiness of women's lives.

Many of women's stories have never been written. They form an oral tradition, passed on from one generation to the next. Sometimes they are just seen as anecdotes about family "characters" and their antics. Sometimes they are teaching stories. They are about having respect, about having decent values, about how to live properly, about how to survive.

Cultures shape stories in different ways, and stories pass on women's consciousness as it has been shaped by cultural, racial, and class experience. Central to women's consciousness, of course, is an understanding of the ways of men. Sometimes we have heard these stories so often we don't think they are important. Then a situation arises, and we need help, and we remember a story because the help we need is embedded in it. We hear the voice of the teller again, and we remember the details. The story is useful. (pp. 39–40)

> Aptheker has gone on to call for "A Gathering of Women" to change the very foundations of society.

What I have been about throughout this book is showing that the dailiness of women's lives structures a different way of knowing and a different way of thinking. The process that comes from this way of knowing has to be at the center of a women's politics, and it has to be at the center of a women's scholarship. This is why I have been drawn to the poetry and to the stories: because they are layered, because more than one truth is represented, because there is ambiguity and paradox. When we work together in coalitions, or on the job, or in academic settings, or in the community, we have to allow for this ambiguity and paradox, respect each other, our cultures, our integrity, our dignity.

As we have pressured against racial and sex discrimination, institutional doors have been opened, however tenuously and with whatever reluctance. Some of us have been allowed in, but nothing about the values of those institutions or their rules of success has changed, whether they be academic, corporate, ecclesiastic, political, medical, or juridical. The point is to change the values and the rules and to change the process by which they are established and enforced. The point is to integrate ideas about love and healing, about balance and connection, about beauty and growing, into our everyday ways of being. We have to believe in the value of our own experiences and in the value of our ways of knowing, our ways of doing things. We have to wrap ourselves in these ways of knowing, to enact daily ceremonies of life.

The desert is a metaphor. For how long women have endured. Like creosote. Waiting for the rains.

We are the rains. (pp. 253–254)

TALES I TELL MY MOTHER

MICHELE ROBERTS is an African American feminist author whose short stories chronicle women's lives. The story excerpted here, "Martha and Mary Raise Consciousness from the Dead," was published in Tales I Tell My Mother.

We carry the memory of childhood like a photo in a locket, fierce and possessive for pain and calm; everybody's past is inviolate, separate, sacrosanct, our heads are different countries with no maps or dictionaries, people walk vast deserts of grief or inhabit walled gardens of joy. "Tell me about your past," I began to urge other women and they to urge me. The women sit in circles, they are passing telegrams along battle lines, telling each other stories that will not put them to sleep, recognizing allies under the disguise of femininity, no longer smuggling ammunition over back garden walls. (p. 72)

CLAIMING AN IDENTITY THEY TAUGHT ME TO DESPISE

MICHELLE CLIFF grew up in Jamaica and New York and was educated in New York and at the University of London. Noted for her essays, articles, lectures, and workshops on racism and feminism, she has written several books including The Land of Look Behind *and* No Telephone to Heaven.

We are still learning to recognize what we see.
Traces erased. Details removed.
Letters sewn into quilts—or burned.
Self-portraits hidden in trunks—or burned.
The perishable nature of so many of our artifacts.

If in our remembrance we find the depth of our history
Will we opt for description only
or choose to ignite the fuse of our knowledge? (pp. 41–42)

In addition to nurturing and healing, writers have focused on other special qualities of women—their resourcefulness, their coping ability, their understanding of complementarity and mutual completion and enhancement, as described in the following passages.

ORDINARY WOMEN/MUJERES COMUNES

ADRIENNE RICH is one of America's foremost poets and feminist theorists. Her works include Of Woman Born: Motherhood as Experience and Institution, *1976;* Blood, Bread, and Poetry: Selected Prose *1979–1985; and many volumes of poetry. This excerpt is from* Ordinary Women/Mujeres Comunes, *1978, edited by S. Miles et al.*

It's the women who cope. . . . The women are salvaging and building what they can, refusing to go quietly, putting up a struggle to the death. Every ordinary woman is extraordinary. The grandmothers, the mothers on the street, the angry housewives, the women in the empty office buildings late at night, the women who never planned this city, never had a thing to say about its priorities, the women whose work is always being undone, whose wars are waged against leadpaint/leaking toilets/rats/roaches/arsonists . . . who still make gardens in flower pots on housing window-sills, worry about holidays, the taste of special foods, rituals for birthing and dying, cleanliness and seemliness, the powerless responsibility for the lives of children, the consequences of sex, the despair and violence of men; women whose labor to create a decent space in an indecent system is perpetually mocked. . . . Women cope. (p. 7)

ENRICHING THE EARTH

MARY CATHERINE BATESON lives in Cambridge, Massachusetts, and serves as Clarence Robinson Professor of Anthropology and English at George Mason University in Fairfax, Virginia. She is the author of With a Daughter's Eye, *a memoir of her parents, Margaret Mead, the noted anthropologist, and Gregory Bateson; of several other books; and of many essays and articles. This selection appeared in* Composing a Life.

The fundamental problem of our society and our species today is to discover a way to flourish that will not be at the expense of some other community or of the biosphere, to replace competition with creative interdependence. At present, we are steadily depleting the planet of resources and biological diversity; the developed world thrives on the poverty of the south. We are in need of an understanding of global relationships that will be not only sustainable but also enriching; it must come to us as a positive challenge, a vision worth fulfilling, not a demand for retrenchment and austerity. This is of course what we do day by day when we refuse to accept the idea that we must reject one part of life to enhance another. Projecting a new vision is artistic; it's a task each of us pursues in composing our lives. One can write songs about sharing; it is hard to write songs about limits.

Solutions to problems often depend on how they are defined. If you look at unfolding lives, you immediately become aware of the processes of redefinition: shelters may come to be seen as constraining walls, interruptions are recognized as moments of fertilization, outrage becomes empowering and freeing. It is possible to look for pattern in seeming disorder and to propose a search for potential benefit in every problem. The strategies we follow are not strategies for victory but for survival and adaptation. Perhaps what we are learning today about the victims of homelessness will provide a clearer vision of the kind of support that every child or adult needs; perhaps celebrating diversity within the African diaspora will answer some of the questions about diversity in American society; perhaps a collection of broken beads can be joined in a necklace of elegance and beauty.

The visions we construct will not be classic pioneer visions of struggle and self-reliance. Rather, they will involve an intricate elaboration of themes of complementarity—forms of mutual completion and enhancement and themes of recognition achieved through loving attention. All the forms of life we encounter—not only colleagues and neighbors, but other species, other cultures, the planet itself—are similar to us and similarly in need of nurture, but there is also a larger whole to which all belong. The health of that larger whole is essential to the health of the parts. Many women raised in male-dominated cultures have to struggle against the impulse to sacrifice their health for the health of the whole, to maintain without dependency. But many men raised in the same traditions have to struggle against pervasive imageries in which their own health or growth is a victory achieved at the expense of the other. We have perhaps a few years in which to combine these. The visions will be both like and unlike familiar religious visions: like, in that they involve the hesitation of reverence before acting to change, the attentive appreciation of the sacredness of what is; unlike, in that they are open. Instead of worshipping ancestors and deities conceived as parents, we must celebrate the mysterious sacredness of that which is still to be born. . . .

. . . Each of us constructs a life that is her own central metaphor for thinking about the world. But of course these lives do not look like parables or allegories. Mostly, they look like ongoing improvisations, quite ordinary sequences of day-to-day events. They continue to unfold. . . . The compositions we create in these times of change are filled with interlocking messages of our commitments and decisions. Each one is a message of possibility. (pp. 239–241)

> Women have magnificently painted their self-portraits as workers in a diversity of occupations. Two of the following profiles appeared in *Women and Work: Photographs and Personal Writings,* 1986. The third is included in Studs Terkel's 1974 treatise, *Working,* in which are recorded hundreds of interviews with workers from all walks of life. These are followed by a poem taking us back to nature—the nature of the earth and the nature of women—in words from an ancient Native American culture, the Anasazi.

CASHIER AND LINE STOCKER

LULÚ CASTAÑEDA, 31, first came to the United States from Mexico when she was 20 years old. She works in an egg packing plant to help support her two children and husband.

My hour to start at work is 5:30 A.M., so I get myself ready at 4:00 A.M. and prepare breakfast for my three children. Then, to begin my shift, I arrive at the egg packing plant and since supposedly I'm the one who speaks English the best, they assigned me to turn on the main machine. Every day I change the number on the computer which marks the boxes which will hold the eggs. The other day I realized that it is a privilege and all the workers on my shift depend on me. It happened that one day I ran out of gas in my car and I was delayed 17 minutes, and when I arrived at the packing plant my co-workers gave me an applause. Nobody had started their work because nobody has the knowledge to start the main machine and the computer. In spite of all, that gave my spirit a new lift. For the first time I felt important in my work.

After starting the main machine and the computer, I go to the line to inspect the eggs, selecting those which are first quality "AA" and separating those which are broken or "cracked." Every day I work one hour as a box girl, and on Wednesdays I work all day as a box girl which is the one day that I do not get dirty with egg. All other days, no matter how much I care for myself, my clothes get covered with egg, including my shoes, and to stand the horrible smell of egg on my clothes. My desperation is to get home before my children and my husband arrive from school and work to take a bath and prepare them dinner. And all this for $3.45 an hour.

In this country I feel like a pioneer because instead of living we survive like the immigrants that we are. Like many other people of different nationalities who have come to the United States in the past, we are all immigrants. Unfortunately, many have forgotten this. In the past, my Black brothers were treated like slaves, and Abraham Lincoln advocated in their behalf and liberated them. Kennedy was killed for the same principles of wanting to help minorities. Martin Luther King is today a hero. And who will advocate for us? How long will we be exploited and humiliated in this same land which belonged to our fathers? Only God knows. He is my hope. With much love to all the world, especially to the women who work in America. (p. 78)

MIDWIFE

JEAN COLLINS is a Certified Nurse Midwife specializing in homebirths.

I never knew what I wanted to be. Remote relatives would ask and expect to have an answer, but at school's end and at the age of 17, I still did not have one. It did not take many days behind a desk for me to decide that wasn't for me, so on my 18th birthday I became a student nurse. In England, it is customary for qualified nurses (who are called State Registered Nurses) to continue their education and specialize in a field of their choice. I chose midwifery and have not regretted my choice.

I landed in the "New World" in 1962 and felt I had taken a step back in time after leaving a country that helped women have babies in their own homes amongst their loved ones. I found myself "helping" women by giving them I.V. injections of scopolamine and restraining them in their beds with side rails and sometimes strapping their hands down. These women would deliver, and maybe two hours later would see their baby. Twenty years later we have come full cycle. Yes, now we truly help mothers have their babies together with family, alert, participating in the birth experience, encouraging involvement and preparation. We can do more . . . many new mothers are not aware of the services available through Certified Nurse Midwives and the dedicated care and educational experience which they offer as an alternative way to have a baby, which is a *natural* process.

Being a nurse-midwife in America is always to be fighting. Fighting for the right to assist parents in a natural process, because some in the medical profession want to make it an unnatural process and invade the maternal body and fetus for tests and procedures. Fighting to stay in the profession without feeling that every day may be your last because an insurance company cannot be found willing to back nurse-midwives as liability coverage.

Midwifery is a profession of extreme emotions; it is working with women and their families to guide them, encourage them and initiate them in the intricacies of childbirth. It is my wish for every pregnant woman I come in contact with to have the most joyous, wonderful obstetrical experience possible. The disappointment in this profession is that obviously, not everyone meets this goal. (p. 147)

PRACTICAL NURSE

CARMELITA LESTER arrived from the West Indies in 1962. She has been a practical nurse for the past five years. "You study everything about humanity, the human body, all the way through. How to give the patient cares, how to make comfortable . . . Most of the time I work seven days."

We're in a private room at a nursing home for the elderly. "Most of them are upper, above middle class. I only work for private patients. Some may have a stroke, some are maybe confused. Some patients have nothing wrong with them, but relatives just bring them and leave them here."

As she knits, she glances tenderly at the old, old woman lying in the bed. "My baby here has cerebral thrombosis. She is ninety-three years old."

I get in this morning about eight-thirty. I shake her, make sure that she was okay. I took her tray, wipe her face, and give her cereal and a cup of orange juice and an egg. She's unable to chew hard foods. You have to give her liquids through a syringe. She's supposed to get two thousand cc per day. If not, it would get dry and she would get a small rash and things like those.

The first thing in the morning, after breakfast, I sponge her and I give her a back rub. And I keep her clean. She's supposed to be turned every two hours. If we don't turn her every two hours, she will have sores. Even though she's asleep, she's got to be turned.

I give her lunch. The trays come up at twelve thirty. I feed her just the same as what I feed her in the morning. In the evening I go to the kitchen and pick up her tray at four o'clock and I do the same thing again. About five thirty I leave here and go home. She stays here from five thirty until eleven at night as floor care, until the night nurse come.

You have to be very, very used to her to detect it that she's having an attack. I go notify that she's having a convulsion, so the nurse come and give her two grains of sodium amytal in her hips. When she gets the needle it will bring down her blood pressure. Because she has these convulsions, her breathing stops, trying to choke. If there's nobody around, she would stifle.

Some days she's awake. Some days she just sleeps. When she's awake she's very alert. Some people believe she isn't, but she knows what's going on. You will hear her voice say something very simple. Other than that, she doesn't say a word. Not since she had that last heavy stroke last year. Before that, she would converse. Now she doesn't converse any more. Oh, she knows what's going on. She's aware. She knows people by the voices. If a man comes in this room, once she hears that voice, I just cannot undress her. (Laughs.) . . . .

The work don't leave my mind. I have been so long with her that it became part of me. In my mind it's always working: "How's she getting along!" I worry what happened to her between those hours before the night nurse report. If I go off on a trip, I'll be talking about her. I'll say, "I wonder what happened to my baby." My girl friend will say, "Which baby are you talking about?" I'll say, "My patient." (Laughs.) I went to Las Vegas. I spent a week there. Every night I called. Because if she has these convulsions. . . .

In America, people doesn't keep their old people at home. At a certain age they put them away in America. In my country, the old people stay in the home until they die. But here, not like that. It's surprising to me. They put them away. The first thing they think of is a nursing home. Some of these people don't need a nursing home. If they have their own bedroom at home, look at television or listen to the radio or they have themselves busy knitting. . . . We all, us foreigners, think about it.

Things that go on here. I've seen many of these patients, they need help, but they don't have enough help. Sometimes they eat and sometimes they don't. Sometimes there's eight hours' wait. Those that can have private nurse, fine. Those that can't suffer. And this is a high-class place. Where *poor* old people. . . . (She shakes her head.) . . .

I feel sorry for everybody who cannot help themselves. For that reason I never rest. As soon as I'm off one case I am on another. I have to sometimes say, "Don't call me for a week." I am so tired. Sometimes I have to leave the house and hide away. They keep me busy, busy, busy all the time. People that I take care of years ago are callin' back and askin' for me. . . .

An elderly person is a return back to babyhood. It give you a feeling how when you were a teenager, you're adult, you think you're strong and gay, and you return back to babyhood. The person doesn't know what's happening. But you take care of the person, you can see the difference. It makes you sad, because if you live long enough, you figure you will be the same.

Postscript: A few months after this conversation, her "baby" died. (pp. 650–655)

AN ANASAZI WOMAN SPEAKS

GINNY ODENBACH teaches gifted students in Wyoming. Her poetry has been published in Westering, Wyoming Writing *1988 and 1989,* Plainswoman, *and* If I Had A Hammer: Women's Work in Poetry, Fiction, and Photographs.

I was here. I came this way.

With the rabbit brush
You dig from your fields
I wove a carrying basket
And worked into it a dark
Design of eagles' claws.
My signature—inked
With sneezeweed dyes.

With the feathers you pluck
From your turkey and burn
I wove a blanket,
A cope to wear when
Winds blow chilly.

With the yucca you ignore
I shod my feet and washed my hair
Weaving sandals from the leaves
And making soapweed suds from the roots.

With the yarrow leaves the wind scatters
I made tea, hot and strong,
To warm and cure and calm.

With the clay beneath your feet
That gumbo which sticks to your boots,
I coiled pots, and mugs,
And sacred feather holders.

With the soft inner bark
Of the juniper, I diapered my baby,
Or crushed it between my hands
To make a nest for the spark
From my fire bow.

I ground red hematite
Between two stones and mixed it
With my honey-colored urine
Then slapped my painty palm
Against the canyon wall, saying,

I was here. I came this way. (pp. 1–2)

And, along with the thread of determination witnessed in the preceding passages, a thread of hope runs throughout the literature on women and work.

"HOPE" IS THE THING WITH FEATHERS

EMILY DICKINSON (1830–1886), reclusive American poet, wrote more than 1700 poems, only a few of which were published during her lifetime. Her solitary life and devotion to her art served as the basis for the play, The Belle of Amherst.

"Hope" is the thing with feathers—
That perches in the soul—
And sings the tune without the words—
And never stops—at all—

And sweetest—in the Gale—is heard—
And sore must be the storm—
That could abash the little Bird—
That kept so many warm—
I've heard it in the chillest land—

And on the strangest Sea—
Yet, never, in Extremity,—
It asked a crumb—of Me. (p. 30)

And a final word on women and work from *Seeds of Light,* a collection of excerpts from the writings of The Mother, published in Pondicherry, India.

We have everyone of us a role to fulfill, a
work to do, a place which we alone can
occupy.

Notes

1. Deena Metzger, "In Her Own Image," *Heresies* I (May 1977): 7.
2. The concept of a women's standpoint is elaborated theoretically in an essay by Nancy Hartsock, "The Feminist Standpoint: Developing the Ground for a Specifically Feminist Historical Materialism," in *Discovering Reality: Feminist Perspectives on Epistemology, Metaphysics, Methodology, and Philosophy of Science,* ed. Sandra Harding and Merrill B. Hintikka (Dordrecht and Boston: D. Reidel, 1983). Hartsock's essay, which I originally read in manuscript in 1980, significantly influenced my ideas in the shaping of this book.

IV

ON HEALTH AND ILLNESS

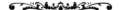

*I*lless is the night-side of life, a more onerous citizen-ship. Everyone who is born holds dual citizenship, in the kingdom of well and in the kingdom of the sick. Although we all prefer to use only the good passport, sooner or later each of us is obliged, at least for a spell, to identify ourselves as citizens of that other place.

Susan Sontag, *Illness as Metaphor,* 1978

Libraries are filled with sections, volumes, and passages on health and illness, the defining concepts of the "health" professions. Within this broad and diverse literature is a multitude of points of view, depending on whether the author has studied, shared, or suffered the health state; has cared for, cared about, or cared with the ill; and has set about to promote health, to conquer disease, to build up the defenses, or to summon the best coping behaviors. There is much to be learned from each of these perspectives, when the mind, body, and soul are invoked in the process, and as long as we eventually come to understand the experience of health care, sickness; disability, recovery, and dying from the inside out.

Other chapters contain primary and secondary themes about attitudes toward health and health care paradigms. This chapter is focused more heavily on illness, that "night-side of life" as Sontag has rightly or wrongly called it, and is followed in the next by selections on healing and recovery.

* * *

Health values, from contrasting global and personal outlooks, have been reflected in the following selections by Henderson and Curtin.

HEALTH IS EVERYBODY'S BUSINESS

VIRGINIA HENDERSON is perhaps this country's best known nurse. Co-author of one of nursing's pioneering textbooks, she has traveled the globe to talk with nurses about the essence of their practice. She worked for 10 years to create the first index to nursing research ever published, and was the prime mover behind the AJN International Nursing Index. Her classic definition of nursing was published in 1958 by the International Council of Nurses and appears here in boldface in these excerpts from a Canadian address given when she received one of her many honorary degrees.

Although it is the fashion—at least in the United States—to talk about "delivery of health services" and the roles of the so-called "professionals," "paraprofessionals," and "indigenous workers" (and nursing personnel fall into all these classes), I believe even these terms fail to stress the most important health concept. They leave out the role of *every man*—the patient or client with whose health the whole argument is concerned.

The first questions to be asked about health in each society are: do its people value human life and do they value health as a quality of life?

When a society such as ours in the United States spends about half of its public funds on its military program, and more of its national income on tobacco, liquor, narcotics, and cosmetics than it does on education or health; when it grossly pollutes its urban environment and distributes its food supplies so unequally that some are hungry—no amount of health care that all health workers combined can "deliver" can be more than the application of a "Band-Aid" to a hemorrhaging artery of the society.

In other words, I am saying that respect for life—and health as a quality of life—is *every man's* business and his most important business.

Collectively, a society must learn how to protect and conserve life, to value a sane mind in a healthy body. The "professionals" and "paraprofessionals" cannot "deliver" health to a society. What health workers do *as citizens* to create a world in which life is conserved and health valued, is more important than their services to those in life's crises and the loveless custodial care they offer the chronically ill and dependent.

Those of us in today's so-called western culture are proud of having extended the average life span by more than 20 years since 1900. Doctors and nurses, the principal "deliverers" of health care, tend to point to this accomplishment as evidence of a successful *system* of medical care. But should they?

The average life span in the United States, for example, has risen from about 50 years in 1900 to about 71 years in 1969, chiefly because infant mortality has dropped dramatically and because children die far less often from infectious diseases in this century than in the last. This drop in infant and child mortality is not so much because doctors and nurses have given good medical and nursing care to infants and children, but because the water they drink and the food they eat is cleaner, and because protective sera, antibiotics, and specific drugs have been developed to protect the young against the pathogenic organisms that in the last century could, and sometimes did, wipe out even large families.

Those who have so greatly increased the life span therefore include not only doctors and nurses, but bacteriologists, chemists, sanitarians, and legislators—all who have identified dangers in the environment, developed controlling agents, and devised protective legislation. Credit is also due biological scientists and educators who have raised the general level of nutrition.

Children of this age talk knowingly about food values, about protecting teeth from decay and, in fact, about health hazards and health practices that were unknown to our great-grandparents. What American school child, for example, would not be aghast to see a doctor spit on his boot, sharpen a knife, wipe it off and lance a boil? Yet, I'm told this is what the country doctor did when he treated the boys in my grandfather's school.

What child of today has not heard the danger of air pollution discussed? A six-year-old friend of mine said to her brother, who was wishing dire disaster on her as a result of a quarrel, "I wish I was pollution and you had to breathe me."

Health care is indeed the business of *every person*. It is the business of the humanist; the philosopher; the priest; the physical, biological or social scientist; the physician to man and beast; the specialist in any branch of therapy; the nurse; the educator; the legislator; and the parent and child.

I believe promotion of health is far more important than the care of the sick. I believe there is more to be gained by helping every man learn how to be healthy than by preparing the most skilled therapists for service to those in crises.

. . . the goal of every health worker should be to help those they serve acquire or regain their independence. The great beauty of medicine, to my mind, is its ethical principle of cooperation as opposed to the industrial principle of competition. A medical worker does not patent and protect his discovery, but freely shares the knowledge and skills he develops with all who can use them.

So, in discussing health and health service, I believe the concept that the *average* man has of health will determine the future. Each of us will strive for what, in our hearts, we value most. We are each the hero or anti-hero of our lives, and the best doctor or the best nurse can only help us reach the goal we set ourselves.

For every health team (another popular term) the patient is really the captain: if he wants to stay sick or die, the rest of the team is nearly impotent. So all health workers are actually assistants to the patient.

Under our western system of medicine, the physician is best prepared to help the patient identify the nature of his illness or handicap and to develop the most effective therapeutic plan or regimen with him, his family, the nurses, the social workers, and others who know the patient and his setting. I hope that some day all countries will have enough physicians to go around; at present the corner druggist is often the poor man's doctor in the United States. Some physicians there—and here too, I believe—would like to turn over certain categories of patients to nurses—specifically, the well child, the chronically ill and aged, and those who must be visited in their homes.

In Russia, physicians' assistants or "feldshers" share responsibility for diagnosing disease and prescribing therapy. Physicians (more than three-quarters of them are women) supervise the feldsher and the nurse. In Russia, nurses have no autonomy and there is no nursing profession. In other countries where western medicine is practiced, the physician is the authority on *cure* and the nurse, the expert on *care*.

In 1934, Ira A. Mackay, then dean of arts and sciences at McGill University in Montreal, spoke of these two essentials: *care* (by the nurse) and *cure* (by the physician). He added, "I do not know which is nobler." I would say, I do not know which is more necessary—or which is more difficult.

I see nursing as a highly complex service demanding broad social experience and a continuing study of the physical, biological, and social sciences. **I believe it is the nurse's unique function to help the individual, sick or well, to carry out those activities contributing to health or its recovery, or to a peaceful death that he would perform unaided if he had the necessary strength, will, or knowledge.** I believe the nurse should fulfill this function in homes, hospitals, schools, industries, prisons, ships, or anywhere else, *whether or not a physician is in attendance.*

This is an elastic definition, as there is infinite variety in the needs of individuals and the circumstances under which they must be met. The nurse may have to help a woman deliver her baby, help pass a tube into an asphyxiated man's windpipe, or even perform a tracheotomy. It includes helping a patient decide whether or not he needs a physician.

If a physician sees a patient and prescribes for him, the nurse must help the patient understand, accept, and carry out the treatment. *Notice I do not say the doctor's orders, for I question a philosophy that allows a physician to give orders to patients or other health workers.*

The nurse's role, as just described, requires her to know the patient; to get inside his skin, assess his physical and emotional needs; to walk for him if he is bedfast; to speak for him if he is mute, or unconscious; to protect him if he is suicidal until she can help him regain his love of life.

When we consider the difficulty of maintaining our own physical and emotional balance, we must see that helping others to do it is indeed a complex service. The nurse must constantly assess the patient's need for strength, will, or knowledge and know how to withdraw this complement of any one of them, so that he gains or regains his independence as soon as possible. The nurse must tailor her service to the patient's chronological and intellectual age, his life experience and setting, his values, his temperament and the limitations imposed by his handicap or illness. Since, in addition, she must help the patient or client understand and carry out the prescribed therapy, the nurse must be a continuing student of medicine, for she can teach only what she knows. (pp. 32–34)

MARIA'S CHOICE

LEAH CURTIN is Editor of Nursing Management *and a prolific writer and speaker on many facets of nursing. This editorial appeared in that journal in 1990.*

How do you take the measure of a man—or a woman? Sister Maria is 75 years old. She is about 4'10" tall and weighs 72 pounds. She has a moderately severe scoliosis of the spine, osteoarthritis and rheumatoid arthritis. She has survived multiple surgeries and a major stroke. Her right shoulder is dislocated. Her jaw has been shattered in a fall—so badly that it cannot be set; she's been mugged seven times at last count.

She suffers more pain than almost anyone I've ever met.

And she's the only one I know who visits a young man convicted of hacking his foster parents to death. Sister Maria started working with street people years ago. Long before it became popular, she struggled to find housing for the homeless. She visits shut-ins, and reads the works of the most contemporary—and often most controversial—theologians. She's usually good for a handout, but she's nobody's fool. If you need food, she's likely to give you a check made out to a local grocery store. Only the uninitiated are deceived by Sister Maria's soft voice and gentle ways: she is a strong woman. A woman of principle. A woman of prayer. A determined woman indeed!

This is her life, and this is how she chooses to live it.

Pain, limited motion, digestive problems, and more pain interfered with her choices, with her living. Finding ways to control the pain and build her strength meant that Maria could go on with her life. It now means that she can work six to eight hours a day, six days a week.

Sister Maria is a woman who "spends" her health. She spends it on things that are more valuable to her than health itself. Sister Maria, and other patients like her, give us a different perspective on health. Health for them is a personal resource, a capacity which enables them to express their values and sense of purpose. By almost any measure, Sister Maria's life is "healthier" than that of many people who are physically fit—and purposeless. She is a woman who chooses to live by her values.

In doing so, she presents her caregivers with difficulties. The stronger she gets, the more she works. The more she works, the greater her stress. The greater her stress, the greater her pain.

She wants to be alert, so she rarely takes pain medications or sleeping pills. The less she sleeps, the weaker she gets. The harder she works, the greater her stress, the tireder she gets, the greater her pain. To keep her going is to keep her working. Often in dangerous areas, or climbing on buses or walking the streets. But "to keep her up and doing" is to enable her to use her life. That not only gives her personal satisfaction but also the opportunity to meet needs she sees as greater than her own.

Lives like Sister Maria's are rare, but are patients like Sister Maria so uncommon? People do value things which enhance the meaning of their lives more than they value health. Few people make health their life goal. Health is a means to an end, not an end in itself. Health is not the goal; living is the goal . . . not life itself, but rather the *living of a life*. Life's "trade-offs" are common—and commonly missed. People often choose to get less sleep than they need, skip a meal, or work long hours under stress in order to do something which is important to them.

Any fair examination of today's health care delivery system will conclude that it focuses on survival. Simplistically put, curing is the goal: an understandable and good but an insufficient end.

Illness and death surround health professionals with pain. Nurses and physicians in particular are "confronted daily with the vulnerability of the human condition, a vulnerability which professional training sensitizes them to detect. Professionals are also confronted daily with the full spectrum of human strength and resilience which they are not as systematically trained to see. Without the ability and skill of seeing the latter, the former may become overwhelming and so painful as to cause people to withdraw and distance, to protect themselves in ways that make them smaller and less alive than they should be."[1]

And patients get efficient, technical service. Sometimes it is even polite. Patient and family are left alone with the illness to follow directions—or not. Usually they go on living, sometimes all the way through life to death. Perhaps because of our perspective, we stay focused on their survival. And we burn out.

The most significant questions health professionals can ask themselves are, "Do I serve *surviving* or *living?*" "Is health really physical fitness or the patient's capacity to respond to her inner direction and her sense of larger purpose?" If so, in daily interaction with patients, the professionals' guiding principle should be the affirmation of the person's life and the support of her growth. The denial of death and the preservation of bodily function are subordinate to the person. Therefore, professionals must consciously acknowledge the context of their work—to see themselves as working in relationship with people rather than as acting on people. Working in relationship *with* people *is caring*. Its function is healing. Indeed, caring is to healing what curing is to survival.

We've already discovered that surviving without healing is appalling. What we have yet to learn is that there is no real curing without caring. Compassionate concern makes people feel that they are understood, not as they seem to be, not as others judge them, but as they are. Every person is important—special, unique—and each one's living is more important than our knowledge, turf and technology. That's the message of caring.

If living is the goal, then our greatest health problem today is that people don't think they are special. We acknowledge their specialness when we share their goals. Thus, even when we may not cure them, our caring still can help heal them. Sister Maria walks the streets again. And she's already been mugged seven times and she'll wear herself out and she'll do as she chooses. That is health. And that, after all, is why we're here. (p. 7)

> Both physiological and pathological processes have been described exquisitely and excruciatingly by medical scientists and clinicians. The nervous system, lupus, tuberculosis, and noscomial infections are the subjects of the following three pieces, illustrating that clinicians and scientists do write good literature. In the fourth, the healer sees himself reflected in the dehumanized, neglected patient.

LIFE ON THE FRONTIERS OF BRAIN SURGERY

DAVID NOONAN is a medical journalist whose work has appeared in Esquire, The New York Times Magazine, Sports Illustrated, *and other publications. He spent five years studying neurologists, neurosurgeons, and their patients; his observations are reflected in the compelling, absorbing book* Neuro—Life on the Front Lines of Neurological Medicine, *from which this excerpt is taken.*

The author begins,

There is nothing in nature as perfect or as powerful as the human nervous system—not the seamless folding of the seasons one into the other; not the rolling, biogenetic mass of the oceans; not the great silent spin of the planets around the sun. The nervous system fires every human act, drives every human moment. It enables man to think and to move, to feel and to wonder, and makes him the dominant life form in the known universe. A charged web that hangs in every human body, its electrochemical circuits carry the elusive spark of life itself. And if that which is human is also somehow divine, then nervous tissue is both the means of the miracle and the miracle itself. Complex beyond man's understanding, the human nervous system is the most sophisticated arrangement of cells that exists.

William Shakespeare at his desk, Albert Einstein at his blackboard, Brooks Robinson at third base, Pablo Casals in concert, Henri Matisse at his easel. These are examples of the human nervous system at work. The composition of *Hamlet,* the formulation of the theory of relativity, the flawless fielding of a line drive, and the rendering of order and beauty in music and painting are all products of the nervous system. Neurons fire in unknown patterns and the world is seen, the universe is understood, man's nature is explored, the ball game is saved . . . . (p. 11)

To approach an understanding of what the nervous system is, what it does, and how it works, you can begin by thinking of it as a kind of membrane. There is a two-way flow of energy through the membrane. On one side is the individual human being, and on the other side, the rest of the world—lovers, accidents, weather, families, meals, beaches, strangers, work, play, beer, the whole deal. Everything that is on the outside gets to the individual through his nervous system; all the various stimuli pass through it. Likewise, the individual gets to the outside world by way of his nervous system; his words and actions pass through it and affect things on the outside. Man is aware of the world outside himself because his nervous system receives and processes all the information that enables him to conclude that the world exists. And man is able to interact with that world because his nervous system provides him with the means to do so. (p. 13)

Two hundred pages later, Noonan concludes his intellectual odyssey:

. . . any attempt to understand human behavior that doesn't take into account the spiritual element of human life is incomplete, a failure of imagination. Even if it is possible to delineate the exact structures, chemicals, and steps involved in the generation of a specific emotion, and someone does it, that won't mean they will have localized the emotion itself. Yes, love is a chemical reaction, but there is more to it than that. There is, I believe, something beyond biology, and it is a factor, somehow, in the function of every living human cell and in every human thought and deed. In a sense, the human nervous system is a complex set of conditions necessary for the existence of the soul. But that is wrong in that is implies a separateness, and there is none. Ultimately, all research into the workings of the nervous system leads to the soul, and all neuroscientists are working in its shadow. Acknowledging the shadow would transform it into a great light, and the work would shine with a new significance, hard science informed by an awareness of the holy unknown.

In the end, I guess, it's a matter of faith. If the future is to be worth the trouble of getting there, that is what it will take—faith in man, faith in the human nervous system, faith in its power, its

perfection, and its instinctive, insatiable need to understand itself. (pp. 218–219)

THE WOLF INSIDE

*JOHN STONE is a cardiologist at Emory University School of
Medicine, and a writer of skill and grace. His writings include
three poetry collections and a book of essays,* In a Country of
Hearts, *from which this excerpt comes.*

Four weeks before she died of a complication of lupus erythema-
tosus, Flannery O'Connor wrote, in a letter dated July 5, 1964,
"The wolf, I'm afraid, is inside tearing up the place. I've been in
the hospital 50 days already this year." By the time of her next
recorded letter three days later, she had received the rite of extreme unction. I never met Flannery O'Connor, but I never see a
patient with lupus now without thinking of those words and of
the woman herself.

The word *lupus* was appropriated whole to the medical vocabulary directly from the Latin meaning "wolf." This autoimmune
system disease affects virtually every organ in the body. About
60 percent of patients will have a red ("erythematous") rash on
the face, over the bridge of the nose, and on the cheeks below the
eyes, in a more or less "butterfly" pattern, a shape similar to the
facial markings of a wolf.

I saw a young woman with lupus today. She doesn't have the rash.
She does have extensive kidney disease and, according to an X
ray, a massively enlarged heart. Hers is a dramatic case: In just
two months, she has gained fifty pounds, all of it water. I go up
to her bed, introduce myself, and shake her hand. As she tells
her story, it's obvious that she is reasonably comfortable. She's
breathing easily, her blood pressure and pulse are good. Since I
was first asked to see her, I have also learned that, despite the
chest X ray, her heart is not enlarged. Rather, the pericardial sac
around it, designed to hold a scant ounce of fluid, has managed to
stretch hugely, accumulating perhaps three quarts of fluid—thus

the enlarged heart shadow on her X ray. She is waterlogged, her tissues swimming in excess fluid that her diseased kidneys cannot excrete. The echocardiograph is like a sonar unit, its echo like the sonogram of a fetus: but instead of a fetus floating within its sac of liquid, there was her heart, normal in size, bobbing and squeezing like a fist.

Her kidney disease is such that she is losing huge amounts of protein in the urine. Normal kidneys are designed to filter the total blood volume selectively many times each day, manufacturing, in the process, several quarts of urine while losing only tiny amounts of protein from the blood that has been filtered. But her kidneys are leaking protein like a sieve. Without that protein to hold the plasma within the blood vessels, she is leaking water into all her tissues, including the pericardial sac. After talking with her at length about her illness, I examine her. A soft, scratchy noise, synchronous with the heartbeat, confirms her inflamed pericardium, one of the problems often seen with lupus. Her legs are grossly swollen. I press my fingers gently into the skin over her shins—the tips of my fingers sink in as though they were poking the soft belly of the puffy little doughboy in the television ad. Several minutes later, as I leave, the deep pits are still there.

Prednisone, a form of cortisone, has been started. The hope is that, in massive doses, the drug will help seal the protein leaks of her kidneys, and that diuretics will mobilize the fifty pounds of excess fluid she has accumulated. The immediate question is whether to use a needle to draw off the fluid from around her heart. The danger is that the fluid will restrict and restrain the heart's action, like the cellophane wrapper on a box of valentine candy, and jeopardize its all-important pumping. I decide we should not attempt to remove the fluid now, reasoning that it will only reaccumulate: the dike has multiple holes in it—the water would only seep back in. The cardiology fellows working with me disagree: they are in favor of the needle. I argue that we should wait for the drugs to work. I worry about her as I go to sleep that night; it is often easier to *do* something, rather than wait, but it's not always best for the patient. We keep a sterile tray, with a long pericardial needle in it, at her bedside, just in case.

Flannery O'Connor had lupus for some fourteen years before she imagined the wolf tearing up the place. The disease had begun, in late 1950, with, as she spelled it, AWTHRITUS. Arthritis, or joint pain, is present in 90 percent of patients with lupus. Just as common is an overwhelming fatigue, often accompanied by fever, loss of appetite, and loss of weight. The exact cause of lupus is uncertain, but it is known that in the course of the disease, the body makes antibodies directed against its own organs, antibodies capable in turn of damaging the organs. The process amounts to a kind of immunological betrayal of its owner by the body, an absolute autoimmune revolution. Lupus is primarily a disease of women (90 percent of cases, with a peak incidence in the childbearing years). Flannery O'Connor's father died of lupus, however, and today, human lymphocyte antigen (HLA) typing, a kind of tissue "matching" that is done for organ transplants, confirms that there may be a genetic predisposition.

New forms of therapy, especially the judicious use of drugs to suppress the immune system, help slow progression of the disease, and also reduce the requirements for steroids, such as cortisone, with their side effects. Though lupus can be serious, the disease is also capricious, with both relapses and remissions: statistically, the majority of patients can look forward to a time when they are relatively free of problems.

Flannery O'Connor had a severe case: clearly, the "wolf" *was* inside. . . .

Dr. Merrill, Flannery's physician, is a former mentor of mine. About twenty years ago, he told me that Flannery's lupus was diagnosed just as more hopeful therapy became available. . . . ACTH, a hormone that causes the body to secrete cortisone, was prescribed for Flannery in the early 1950s. The effect of ACTH (and cortisone, which she took later) is to blunt the body's response to the turncoat antibodies of lupus. The drugs worked—at a price. ACTH and cortisone can have significant side effects: thinning of bone (osteoporosis); loss of muscle strength; a moonlike shape to the face; exacerbation of duodenal ulcers; altered metabolism; increased susceptibility to infections; mood changes, ranging from a feeling of well-being to depression and even psychosis.

Flannery was well aware of the side effects as she wrote: "My dose of prednisone had been cut in half on Dr. Merrill's orders because the nitrogen content of the blood has increased by a third. So far as I can see, the medicine and the disease run neck & neck to kill you." But she felt better on the medications. In 1960, after ten years on steroids, she wrote that "as Dr. Merrill says, it is better to be alive with joint trouble than dead without it. Amen."

Over the next week, as I see my own young lupus patient, I can tell, thank God and prednisone, she is improving. She has lost more than thirty pounds, all of it water. The pericardial fluid has diminished—her echo looks better. She's going to make it. And she gives me a tired, heroic smile.

Heroic is, I think, the word for Flannery O'Connor too. When the disease struck her, she was twenty-five, a graduate of the Iowa Writers' Workshop, a fledgling writer just beginning to make a name for herself. Despite the wolf, the next fourteen years were productive ones for her. She won three O. Henry first prizes; the National Book Award came posthumously, in 1971. Many of her best short stories were written during these years: "A Good Man Is Hard to Find" in 1953; "Good Country People" in 1955; "Everything That Rises Must Converge" in 1961; "Revelation" in the spring of 1964, just months before she died.

Flannery O'Connor knew at least two kinds of isolation—that required by her craft and that imposed by her illness. Listen to her in 1956: "I have never been anywhere but sick. In a sense sickness is a place, more instructive than a long trip to Europe, and it's always a place where there's no company, where nobody can follow." Of course, in a metaphorical sense, Flannery O'Connor never stopped traveling. And the joy of discovery kept her at the typewriter. From one of the earliest of her collected letters (July 21, 1948), there is evidence that the process of writing was, for her, journey enough: "I have to write to discover what I am doing. Like the old lady, I don't know so well what I think until I see what I say."

Flannery O'Connor *endured* . . . despite the lupus. That she weathered the devastating side effects of ACTH and cortisone, continuing to write, slowly, painfully, to find out exactly what she *did* think, makes her a heroine to me. But then, many of my patients seem heroic to me, especially the ones with chronic illnesses.

Through its Latin root, the word *doctor* means "teacher"; but very often it is the patient who does the teaching, especially when the lesson is one in courage. It's one thing to have an acute, limited illness, to pass the bloody agonizing kidney stone and be done with it; it's quite another to go to sleep with pain, to dream that it's gone, then wake back up to the same pain waiting like a wild beast at the foot of your bed. And to persevere despite the pain, feeling it flow like electricity out of your forearms along your sore wrists and out to your stiff fingers to discover precisely how the twenty-six letters of the alphabet plan to marry *this* time.

Lupus betrayed Flannery O'Connor like a sophisticated Trojan horse, one with a wolf inside. Once within the body's gates, the enemy was everywhere. Still, she prevailed, even if it was only until her thirty-ninth year. And her life and words are a study in keeping on keeping on. It is in that spirit that I move to the next patient. (pp. 59–64)

OCTOBER

JAMES H. BUCHANAN, medical writer and ethicist, holds a doctorate in philosophy with an emphasis on epistemology and the relationship between perception and neurophysiology. The compelling narratives that form Patient Encounters: The Experience of Disease *grew from journal entries based on his experiences with patients who suffered from various disorders. One of the most powerful is excerpted here.*

Later, the day would break clean and brilliant across the Johns Hopkins University Hospital. But now it was still dark and rather cool for September 15, 1938. High up, against the darkness, there was at least one room illuminated by the vigil of family members waiting for a loved one to die. For the past three days, their brother, their son, their friend had lain in a coma from exploratory brain surgery. At first he rallied, but then yesterday—or was it the day before?—the old and subtle enemies of pneumonia and pulmonary infection had sought him out and found him without defenses. Now it was almost 6:30 A.M. on a Thursday morning, and within minutes Thomas Wolfe would be dead. Had he lived but another eighteen days, he would still have only been thirty-eight years old. How strange that death should find him there, in that place which also had claimed his father.

When the details of his death became known, some would claim that all of his genius, all of his power and eloquence were simply the insanity of a diseased brain seeking to free itself from its misery. Cruel? Yes, of course, certainly cruel. But far more strange than cruel. How strange to reduce a human spirit to the agony it endured. How strange to denounce in a single judgment all that was rich, poetic, glorious, and supremely human to the erratic cell division of a pathological process. Such denouncements, in effect, deny that the artist has seen beauty and claim instead that he has simply suffered madness.

Others, however, would hear of his death and feel the earth shudder for just a moment. They mourned for him, but far more for themselves and for the lost words, the beautiful phrases, and the powerful insights that had now disappeared from history. And still others cared little about his death or his life because he meant nothing to them, and they felt no change in the climate or condition of the earth.

What shall we make of an artist's death? After all, is there anything to be made of it at all? He is not special or different from other men who have lived and suffered in similar ways. Does the artist enjoy any special privileges that should make him immune to destruction? Why then should we be surprised or even disturbed by his death? Is the world any better for having entertained briefly Chaucer, Shakespeare, Michelangelo, Dante, Eliot, and Wolfe? Their words, their works were beautiful to behold, but what of that? They often agonized more and certainly spoke more about their agony and in finer words, but what of that? They thought about their lives and often about their deaths, but we have also seen what they have seen and has it made us any better? So what of all this?

Perhaps it is true that these artists are howling madmen who overexaggerate their suffering and break vows of silence that the rest of us choose to keep sacred. Perhaps too much can be made of an artist's death in September. He wrote fine words, yes, and saw great things, yes, but what of all that for us who have seen the same and remained silent?

Tuberculosis has always been a disease of artists. One cannot think of Keats, of Chopin and fail to associate the suffering of their lives with the suffering of their art. Pale, wan, and emaciated from the power of their remarkable gifts, those who create seem ultimately to be destroyed by internal engines too powerful to be contained within the slender frame of the poet. It is a most romantic notion, but appropriately so when used to describe artists such as Keats, Chopin, and Wolfe.

However, tuberculosis is not simply of the lungs or of the bone or of the brain, but rather of each and all of these. It is especially fond of seeking residence in the great dynamic centers of our lives: where we think or where we breathe or even in the skeletal cement that holds us together. For herein it can do what it does best: consume. Tuberculosis is a disease which devours, consumes, and finally digests its victim, and in this regard it is a disease much like cancer. But the latter is a madness gone wild which consumes without reason and without plan; whereas, tuberculosis is a madness in perfect control of itself. So true is this that the disease may wait patiently in remissive tissue for years until some sudden spark of inspiration causes it to roam in search of new histological territories. Certainly this was true of Thomas Wolfe that ill-begotten summer of 1938.

Wolfe was invited to speak at Purdue University on May 19, 1938. It was the usual academic affair with professors from each department waiting to meet him and get his autograph. After his talk at Purdue, he traveled to Chicago, and then a few days later he boarded a sleek and powerful train—the Burlington Zephyr— and left for Denver with the claim that both coach bars on board would be dry before he arrived. From Denver, he went to Portland and from Portland to Seattle. His arrival and eventual return to Seattle were interrupted by a two-week hiatus in which he traveled with two other companions to eleven parks in the western states. Back in Seattle, he departed once again for Vancouver on the steamer *Princess Kathleen.* But in transit he caught a very bad cold and shortly thereafter returned to Seattle. Within days, Wolfe's cold had turned into pneumonia, and at the urging of friends he entered a private hospital for treatment. Despite three days of high fever and alarming symptoms, Wolfe considered himself to be out of danger by July 15. In fact, however, the danger was just beginning, and in his euphoria at being cured of the pneumonia he failed to recognize an even more insidious enemy at work.

There are diseases whose power and fury overwhelm the victim with a savage intensity. They neither court nor seduce nor beckon with sly and retiring ways but instead rape, pillage, and plunder what few reserves remain. But tuberculosis is not one of these. Rather, it toys, experiments, and tantalizes in the most unpredictable ways. There are days when you seem almost symptom free and days as well when your very bones and tissues are rent asunder by pain of indescribable proportions. It is a strange illness which seems either to sleep or to roam with restless energy as it did with Thomas Wolfe that summer of 1938. For within him, the lesions of a past tubercular scarring began to blossom once again very much as a rose in springtime responds to warmth and soil and moisture by bursting forth. Breaking all bounds of propriety and limitation, the tubercular seeding freed itself from the confines of the lungs, sought out the large bronchial blood vessels, and migrated in dozens of different directions.

There exists an invisible but extremely powerful blood-brain barrier which captures most illnesses within its entanglements before they can invade that closed casket of thoughts, ideas, and feelings. Even the great viral infections are usually stopped by this overseer which carefully inquires into the precise credentials of each traveler. But tuberculosis can be so very charming, so innocent and pure of malevolent intentions that even this most powerful governor is often deceived and thereby allows to pass a Trojan horse of insidious design which masquerades as another. Climbing slowly from lungs to brain, the metastatic foci are in search of fertile ground in which to raise their violent young. They pass by the smooth, pink cardiac tissue and mount even beyond the airy, wispy stretch of alveoli, reaching higher, ever higher. Quickly traveling beyond the most inviting carotid arteries—tempted but not seduced by their loveliness—even beyond the fierce, powerful sternocleidomastoid muscles and still yet beyond the white, barren starkness of mastoid and maxillary bone, the tubercles pursue their mission of metaplasia. They wish to transform, to claim healthy tissue into the geography of their own domain. Finally, finally, there is a landmark seen in the distance. There, wrapped and coiled about itself like an endless snake, entwine the cerebral twists of puffy gray cortex. . . . (pp. 70–74)

———————

Dear God, the headaches were terrible in their awful intensity! Starting now at the temple points and then expanding outward like a Chinese fan, they curled and coiled and cantilevered across the brow, down the neck and seemed to vibrate all the cranial nerves from trigeminal to glossopharyngeal. But more than the pain, far more than simply the agony of it all was the terrific and terrible pressure that seemed to verge on the explosion or implosion of the gentle tissues so compressed. And with each and every pulsation of his heart, there emanated a wave of such profound pain and nausea that he thought he could barely stand the passing moments. Every diastole and every corresponding systole produced a contrapuntal expansion and contraction of the nauseating, pressurized pain. It was intolerable; it was unendurable! Dear God, if only it would stop for just a few moments. But neither sleep nor drugs distracted its intensity.

On August 12 the headaches began in earnest, and they did not depart until Wolfe died thirty-four days later. The agony of those thirty-four days was unceasing. On the afternoon of the same day,

Wolfe wrote to his former friend and editor at Scribner's, Maxwell Perkins (*Editor to Author,* p. 141):

> *Dear Max:*
>
> *I'm sneaking this against orders—but "I've got a hunch"—and I wanted to write these words to you.*
>
> *I've made a long voyage and been to a strange country, and I've seen the dark man very close; and I don't think I was too much afraid of him, but so much mortality still clings to me—I wanted desperately to live and still do and I thought about all of you 1000 times, and wanted to see you all again, and there was the impossible anguish and regret of all the work I had not done, of all the work I had to do—and I know now I'm just a grain of dust, and I feel as if a great window has been opened on life I did not know about before—and if I come through this, I hope to God I am a better man, and in some strange way I can't explain, I know I am a deeper and wiser one. If I get on my feet and out of here, it will be months before I head back, but if I get on my feet, I'll come back.*
>
> *Whatever happens—I had this "hunch" and wanted to write you and tell you, no matter what happens or has happened, I shall always think of you and feel about you the way it was the 4th of July 3 yrs. ago when you met me at the boat, and we went out on the cafe on the river and had a drink and later went on top of the tall building and all the strangeness and glory and the power of life and of the city were below.*
>
>

Yours always,
Tom

Perkins trembled when he read the letter, for it was a certain death knell rung by the one whose passing it would announce. . . . (pp. 75–76)

———————

The brain is such a strange organ! It is the first to sense danger elsewhere but the very last to recognize such trauma within itself. The eyes, the ears, and all the cavities of the brain are the sentinels that monitor disorder and chaos everywhere else but are blinded to such confusion within themselves. The eye sees but cannot see itself seeing. The ear hears but cannot discern the subtle tones of its own hearing. The brain feels the body feeling but is anesthetized to feeling itself. Why? Why does it choose to operate according to such contradictory directives? Would it overwhelm itself with feeling if it also felt? Would the eye blind itself with seeing, or the ear become deaf to hearing, if just this additional ingredient of self-consciousness were added to an already overburdened set of responsibilities? Held captive by a bony cranium which permits neither retreat nor advance, the brain is riveted in place. It cannot expand, neither can it contract, but remains a fruit whose outer seed prohibits internal blossoms. Consequently, every swelling, every shift, every movement is experienced not as pain but as pressure. And as the pressure increases, so does it intimidate and pester everything that has the vanity of feeling: eyes, muscles, meninges, and nerves of every length and caliber. . . . (p. 77)

<hr />

Thomas Wolfe died at 6:30 A.M. Thursday morning . . . not of tuberculosis but of pneumonia. The great diseases—cancer, heart dysfunction, tuberculosis—are rarely the cause of our death, although they are certainly the cause of our suffering. Rather, it is the nosocomial infections caused by *Klebsiella, Proteus, Candida,* or *Enterobacter* that wait in silent expectation of our weakened condition. With a genius and a planning all their own, these opportunistic infections reside within the safe confines of hospitals and sickrooms where the visitor seeking an angel of death obediently comes to them. Their mission is not to degrade, degenerate, or decompose living tissues—this heavy work is left for the catastrophic diseases such as lymphatic leukemia, hypogammaglobulinemia, myeloma, or macroglobulinemia—but rather to whisper the solace and sanctuary of death to the tortured and the damned. Their mission, to that end, is noble, kind, and aristocratic, and even their beautiful names suggest such an elevated office: *Norcardia, Aspergillus, Cryptococcus,* and *Histoplasma.* Let us therefore honor and respect these merciful diseases of the night which reach out in the most divine hours of our lives to touch us with forgiveness and charity. With death now so near, they are truly the only friends remaining who know our suffering and will relieve us of it. For years they have prepared themselves for this exalted moment in our lives. Generations upon generations of pneumococcal, staphylococcal, or pneumocystic pneumonias have strengthened and armored themselves against all antibacterial treatments. Millions have been sacrificed in order to insure this most powerful resistance to any known treatment, and now they are prepared to whisper sweet words of reassurance and comfort to this most lonely one sequestered by his immense suffering. We shall sing to them praises of thanksgiving and adoration, for they remember us when others have forgotten; they know our deep misery and carefully administer the proper antidote; they open the only door through which our feeble bodies may now walk. Searching, ever searching, the corridors and alleyways of the sterile environment for their brothers and sisters, they found Thomas Wolfe that desperate day in September. He was afraid, huddled against himself with terrible tubercular storms raging within, and they were gentler, kinder, yes, even more merciful than anyone had ever been before. With extraordinary skill, they begin to fill his pleural cavities with fluids and exudates of their peculiar composition.

One simply drowns! It is not unpleasant; it is not painful or even frightening if one will simply allow these merciful angels to do what they do best. Higher and higher the bacteremic fluids rise within the pleural cavities, and one feels dizzy, perhaps even a bit giddy, as the tide of suffocation encapsulates from within rather than without. The heart begins to triphammer its octaval concordance, and the mucosal tissues blush blue and cyanotic with consent. The skin sweats profusely in a futile effort to empty these immense fluids, while cacophonous disharmonies of rales and asymphonic breaths protest the inevitability of their eventual silence. The body becomes a metabolic oven of blast-furnace temperatures rising now from 100 to 102 to 105 and beyond. The thermostat melts and can no longer monitor itself as cardiac arrhythmia establishes its delirious cadence. But then, suddenly, there is silence, cessation, and an end to it all. Having risen to the crest of a metabolic high, one simply falls through the center of gravity to a hollow vortex and beyond. It was good, it was merciful and even kind that Thomas Wolfe's immense suffering for the past two months should so end in the peace and grace of nothingness. . . .

All death, finally, is the result of anoxia. All death, finally, issues in the deprivation of oxygen without which the fragile, delicate brain suffocates. Whether cancer or heart disease or lung tumor or liver dysfunction was the catalytic factor that resulted in anoxia is irrelevant. In the end, life reduces to these most elementary biological terms: a grave dependency upon the vital but invisible oxygen molecules to which the brain is so addicted that even gradual withdrawal is at once fatal. . . . In every case, the result is the same: instant and immediate death. Of course, the predisposing cause is always another factor such as a tumor, bacteria, virus, or functional disorder. But these are never the truth of the matter. No, the truth of life is that only air—simple, elementary, invisible air—stands between life and death.

There is neither poetry nor prose to these facts. In its simplest terms, it means that a veil of the most delicate gossamer separates us from an envelope of darkness and nonbeing. It means that every great thought, every cruel art and practice, every wicked motivation, and every sublime inspiration, as well as every small lust and every great triumph of man, rests upon this slender axis of simply breathing air. It means that every beautiful face, every soft and seductive body in the night, every great genius that ever lived and every monster of history, every fool, every dunce, every sorrowful and every joyful life did so only because of air. It means that air, simple, invisible air, is the tie that binds every great and every small man, every lover and every hater, every master and every slave of history into a brotherhood that can be broken only by death. How strange! How strange that air should have this power.

Death is decompression; it is the evaporation and liquefaction of all that unifies, integrates, and solidifies us. Therefore, all that is noble, good, sacred, monstrous, and marvelous about us stands continually upon the verge of evaporation; and since this decompression occurs instantaneously, it will dissolve without warning all that you thought was proud, noble, and secure about yourself.

So in the end—or so it seems—there is no actual end. That is, there is no transition or gradual habituation of life to death. No, one does not really suffer or waste away. Rather, one evaporates into the thinnest air from whence one came and leaves merely a husk of some degree or dimension behind. Where, after all, is the poetry or prose, the sense or meaning, the nobility or tragedy of it?

Thomas Wolfe's head had been shaved to permit brain surgery, and he had lost over fifty pounds throughout his illness. This, along with the pale and waxen quality by which death always announces its domination, transformed him into a preposterous caricature of his former self. Of course, what is truly absurd is not that he was so transformed from life into death but rather the human efforts made to transform him back again. Why do we cling with such ferocious pride to the effigies we make of ourselves?

The Wolfe family returned to Asheville, North Carolina, with his body, and he was buried in Riverside Cemetery beside his father. Should one visit the grave today and seek to find beneath the clover and grass some energy yet remaining of that intense dynamo of life, there is none. Should one look carefully, even searchingly, at the trees, the ground, the flowers for some evidence that here rests a poet and not a mere man, there is none. Should one look for a sign, a symbol, or an apparition of what was unique about him, there is none. This could well be the grave of a tired old lady, of a young child, of a farmer, butcher, doctor, or potter. It could contain the remains of a violent or lustful or gentle or maddened soul. The earth is inscrutable and most mysterious about the secrets it contains. Of course, it is poetic, most romantic to believe that herein will be found something special or unique that marked and qualified his death just as it enunciated his life. But no, there is nothing of the sort here among these flowers and clover and grass. Rather, there are only the endless rows of gravestone upon gravestone with each much like the other and only this peculiar combination of vowels and consonants—Thomas Wolfe—which separates the one from the other. And yet even that is an illusion. The truth is that there is no diameter which distinguishes the dead from one another. Life enunciates, individuates by contours, faces, and body surfaces that differentiate the living from one another. But death knows no such differences since to die is precisely to lose all such individuality and separation. Death is the evaporation of uniqueness and separateness into universality, collectivity, and anonymity.

The poet, the artist, the writer seeks exactly to distinguish himself or herself through the style and personality of his or her craft. In no other profession is the glorification of self so approved and applauded. And yet nature despises such celebrations and abuses the one who insists upon these triumphs. Thus, he suffers not because he must but rather because he counts individuality higher than happiness and contentment. In so disrupting the center-gravity of unity and integration, nature revenges this hubris by a decompression which brings about its very opposite. (pp. 82–86)

ON DEEPER REFLECTION

GREG A. SACHS is a Chicago physician who contributed this "A Piece of My Mind" article to the Journal of the American Medical Association.

Mrs Smith had been transferred to our geriatrics and chronic disease ward the preceding afternoon while I had been away at clinic. Her lengthy record looked painfully similar to so many others I had read during the first five months of my geriatrics fellowship. She was 87 years old. The chart listed her diagnoses as dementia, pressure sores, incontinence, diabetes, anemia, malnutrition, and multiple fractures. The history did not describe the fractures. Perhaps someone had decided that such detail was not required, given all of Mrs Smith's other problems.

She was bedridden, responsive only to painful stimuli. A Foley catheter and a gastrostomy feeding tube were in place. Her albumin level was 1.5. She had been in this state for at least three months, as she had been in the transferring hospital for that long after being admitted there in a hypoglycemic coma. The head nurse informed me that Mrs Smith was hypothermic.

"The temperature is 94.8 rectally," the ward nurse said as I entered Mrs Smith's room. She cried out, seemingly in pain, as the nurse turned her on her left side. The rest of her vital signs were surprisingly normal, although she was slightly tacypneic. She had many pressure sores, including large ones on both heels that were still covered by thick, black eschar.

"My name is Dr Sachs, Mrs Smith," I introduced myself. I placed a hopefully reassuring hand on the patient's shoulder. Her skin was cool and clammy. She cried out as I touched her. "I'm one of the doctors here on the floor," I said. "I'm going to examine you to see what we can do to help you feel better." I began to examine an open wound over her right trochanter. I wondered why her previous physicians had bothered to débride this wound while allowing the sores on her heels to retain their ugly, black covering. The hip sore was two by three centimeters on the surface but was extensively undermined.

As I moved forward to look deeper into the sore, I thought I saw movement within the wound. I immediately felt repulsed and feared that there might be maggots in this poor woman's hip. I saw no organisms, the wound looked clean, and there was a strange clearness in the center of the crater. I took a deep breath and looked again at the ulcer. Once more I noted movement within the sore. This time the movement paralleled my own motions. I moved closer and peered deeper into the cavity. Right in the center, in the deepest portion of the wound, I saw my own reflection staring back at me.

Again I looked to convince myself that I was indeed seeing my own reflection, moving in the wound as I moved outside of it. I moved the opening in the skin back and forth to see more of the tissues below. As more was revealed, it dawned on me that I was seeing myself in Mrs Smith's hip prosthesis, the shiny artificial head of her femur mirroring the image of my face. With her immobility, malnutrition, anemia, and infection, this sore would never heal. I took one more look at myself and then left the room.

Seeing oneself in a pressure sore is a stark and frightening vision, disturbing on many levels. In addition to the grotesque wound and personal reflection, it seemed to mirror the topsy-turvy medical care given to many such patients. Mrs Smith came from a hospital where she received mechanical ventilation for a respiratory arrest suffered when she was hypoglycemic. She had pleural effusions tapped and analyzed and innumerable laboratory tests performed. Yet she lay long enough without being turned for all the tissue between her skin and bones to necrotize.

It is sad that somewhere in the course of a dementing process Mrs Smith lost many of the characteristics that most of us associate with meaningful adult human life. It is sadder still that she received medical treatment that forgot about her as a human being.

It is fitting to have seen myself literally within Mrs Smith and now to carry a vivid memory of her within me. It is a sharp reminder that I am always inside patients like Mrs Smith and that they are always inside me; all of us are part of the human community, no matter how demented, contracted, or incontinent. Debilitated and dependent patients need us to reach out and care for them most when we are starting to push them away. It is our distancing of ourselves from these people that is the true dehumanizing act.

Frequently, I have caught myself praying that I would not contract any of the horrible diseases I saw during residency. Now, mostly, I pray, "Please, dear Lord, do not let me die with pressure sores." (p. 2145)

Writers have described the struggle, the isolation, and the betrayal felt when the senses are lost or diminished. Presented here are pieces of compelling literature about deafness and blindness.

BEETHOVEN'S QUIET MISERY

LUDWIG VAN BEETHOVEN wrote this open letter on October 6, 1802, at age 32. It was taken from the "Heiligenstadt Testament," and appeared in The Letters of Beethoven, *edited by Emily Anderson. The composer, who began losing his hearing in his late 20s, produced many of his greatest works when he was completely deaf.*

O my fellow men, who consider me or describe me as unfriendly, peevish, or even misanthropic, how greatly do you wrong me. For you do not know the secret reason why I appear to you to be so. Ever since my childhood my heart and soul have been imbued with the tender feeling of goodwill; and I have always been ready to perform even great actions. But just think, for the last six years I have been afflicted with an incurable complaint which has been made worse by incompetent doctors. From year to year my hopes of being cured have gradually been shattered and finally I have been forced to accept the prospect of a *permanent infirmity* (the curing of which may perhaps take years or may even prove to be impossible). Though endowed with a passionate and lively temperament and even fond of the distractions offered by society I was soon obliged to seclude myself and live in solitude. If at times I decided just to ignore my infirmity, alas! how cruelly was I then driven back by the intensified sad experience of my poor hearing. Yet I could not bring myself to say to people: "Speak up, shout, for I am deaf." Alas! how could I possibly refer to the impairing *of a sense* which in me should be more perfectly developed than in other people, a sense which at one time I possessed in the greatest perfection, even to a degree of perfection such as assuredly few in my profession possess or have ever possessed—Oh, I cannot do it; so forgive me, if you ever see me withdrawing from your company which I used to enjoy. Moreover my misfortune pains me doubly, inasmuch as it leads to my being misjudged. For me there can be no relaxation in human society, no refined conversations, no mutual confidences. I must live quite alone and may creep into society only as often as sheer necessity demands; I must live like an outcast. If I appear in company I am overcome by a burning anxiety, a fear that I am running the risk of letting people notice my condition—And that has been my experience during the last six months which I have spent in the country. My sensible doctor by suggesting that I should spare my hearing as much as possible has more or less encouraged my present natural inclination, though indeed when carried away now and then by my instinctive desire for human society, I have let myself be tempted to seek it. But how humiliated I have felt if somebody standing beside me heard the sound of a flute in the distance and *I heard nothing,* or if somebody heard *a shepherd sing* and again I heard nothing—Such experiences almost made me despair, and I was on the point of putting an end to my life—The only thing that held me back was *my art.* For indeed it seemed to me impossible to leave this world before I had produced all the works that I felt the urge to compose; and thus I have dragged on this miserable existence—a truly miserable existence, seeing that I have such a sensitive body that any fairly sudden change can plunge me from the best spirits into the worst of humours—*Patience,* that is the virtue, I am told, which I must now choose for my guide; and I now possess it—I hope that I shall persist in my resolve to endure to the end, until it pleases the Parcae [Fates] to cut the thread; perhaps my condition will improve, perhaps not; at any rate I am now resigned. (p. 90)

On His Blindness

JOHN MILTON (1608–1674) was an English poet best known for his epic poems, Paradise Lost *and* Paradise Regained.

When I consider how my light is spent
Ere half my days in this dark world and wide,
And that one talent which is death to hide
Lodged with me useless, though my soul more bent
To serve therewith my Maker, and present
My true account, lest he returning chide,
"Doth God exact day-labour, light denied?"
I fondly ask. But Patience, to prevent
That murmur, soon replies, "God doth not need
Either man's work or his own gifts. Who best
Bear his mild yoke, they serve him best. His state
Is kingly: thousands at his bidding speed,

And post o'er land and ocean without rest;
They also serve who only stand and wait."

Experiencing illness is described in the following pieces about cancer and a disease of unknown etiology.

THE UNIVERSE OF THE ILL

MAX LERNER describes himself as a writer and a teacher, having taught at Brandeis, Sarah Lawrence, Williams, and Notre Dame. Author of many books, he wrote Wrestling with the Angel, *from which this selection is taken, after his bouts with cancer and heart disease. He writes a syndicated column for the Los Angeles Times Syndicate, and lives in New York City and Long Island.*

You enter a hospital with the burden of your fears and hopes. You leave it with both still there but in a very different combination. That's why, if you sit watching at the reception office, the patients entering show a gray sameness of anxiety and depression. If you watch at the departure door the lucky ones seem to be emerging from a dark tunnel.

Jenny came and signed out for me and I went down in the traditional wheelchair to the hospital exit. These entries, exits and re-entries, which go with the territory of the ill, were to become a too familiar ritual in my succession of hospital surgeries and treatments.

I was shaky in the cab. I gazed at the normal world of cars and shopkeepers and young women wheeling their baby carriages, and lovers with their arms entwined, much as a newly released prisoner stares at the normal world from which he was cut off.

Home was bittersweet, sweet because it was our territory, Jenny's and mine, bitter because I didn't know when I would see it again. So I caressed the much read and loved books and gazed out of our windows at the East River tugboats pushing the ships and barges. The scene was a symbol for me of the stream of experience running through our lives. I found my favorite chair, savored the food, riffled through my mail and magazines, and felt for a fleeting moment in touch again with the universe of the well.

I clung to my ties with that universe. I was cancer-ridden, my weight had dropped sharply, and I got little reassurance from any mirror. The "I" that stared back at me was startlingly different from the "I" in the California photo, the one with my arms stretched to the sky, lifting the bars.

In most of our lives we take Time with a capital T for granted, but my illness left me with a sharp consciousness of its implacable brevity. I would take my chances on my cancer in a timeless universe. In my present state I desperately wanted Time to stand still.

It didn't. So I retraversed my choices and found little that was new. Yet I did find one perspective that might clarify things. It was the matter of irreversibility. The chemotherapy might not work, but if I didn't try it now I would never know—and later it might be too late. Without it, including all its negatives, the tumor might grow with no redress. The hackneyed adage was true after all: "Better safe than sorry!"

There wasn't the same urgency about the alternative, or "adjunctive," therapies. I could still use them to supplement the chemotherapy but not the other way around. Moreover, I could apply them myself. I wouldn't need a hospital for that. Wherever I found myself I could use my own affirmations.

Looking back at it from the safer haven of today, all this seems pretty self-evident. But earlier it wasn't. I had to work it out within myself but I did it more clearly in the quiet of my home, seeking a larger frame and strategy, a wider knowing.

I was learning the arts of being ill. "If Contingency is King," I wrote later in my journal, "then in his Kingdom you have to live from day to day at his will."

So after an easeful week at home I came back to the hospital and started my protocol. The drug of choice—actually of non-choice—assigned to me was Adriamycin, combined with Cytoxan and two other drugs. I got weighed and measured so that Dr. Silver could calculate how much to give me. Too little and the killer cells would gain on me, too much and it would savage my system.

The doctor administering it had to become a master of equilibration. Fortunately for me, as Jerry had known in choosing him, Dick Silver* had exactly the right quality of concentration on the individual case.

That the power to heal and the power to kill are often combined is a paradox that goes deep to the nature of things. In the anthropology of medicine we know that the primitive medicine man had control over charms and poisons together. In Elizabethan England the apothecary and chemist were the only physicians available to most. Modern chemotherapy builds on basic nineteenth- and twentieth-century research, which made biochemistry the heart of our pharmacological armory. As literary associations rumbled through my mind I found it ironic that someone who had all but flunked chemistry should be staking his life on the proposition that a mixture of chemical molecules was possessed of the potency to kill the killer cells before they killed him.

It was a wager in the purest form, not on the fights or horses but on life itself. The celebrator of Broadway sporting life, Damon Runyan, calculated that "all life is six-to-five against." It was meant cynically, but I would have gladly settled for the odds. I gathered that in my coming chemical wager, despite my being bolstered by the weight of modern medical technology, the odds were more steeply against me.

I had been much taken by Tennyson's *Idylls of the King.* I now half expected Merlin, maguslike, to enter with the cup. If I was to drink the healing potion I should have liked it in a silver chalice, preceded by a flourish of trumpets. Instead there came a very businesslike nurse pushing a trolley mounted with a large inverted bottle. I didn't drink the potion, which was fed into my system intravenously through a needle inserted in my wrist. Lying in bed I used to watch the clockwork drip-drip of the liquid which slowly, efficiently—along with my other drugs—was transforming my interior into a chemical vat.

During much of my early illness I felt split into two selves, one the "sick" self I had to live *with,* the other the "normal" one I was

---

*Jerry was Lerner's primary physician, Dick Silver was his oncologist.

trying to live *by*. I knew I had in some way to integrate them, but that was not easily done. A war was being waged between them until the healing could set in and the sick self could become the jumping-off point toward a new balance. I discovered ruefully that there is no "norm" to which the sick self struggles to "return." We live life forward, however perilously, although we retrace it backward, and after each travail we are lucky if we achieve a new equilibrium, never quite the one we left behind.

I began to see this as the essential nature of the healing process, by whatever agents it takes place—doctors, drugs, self, or all three together. Accordingly, toward the end of my chemotherapy, I wrote a reflective note in my journal workbook:

> *November 7, 1983   The chemotherapy enables the organism to find a new dynamic, which leads to a new equilibrium. . . . While cancer cells are dividing, others are now resisting them, in battle. Out of that resistance a new equilibrium shows itself which we call a "remission." . . . Illness is the failure of the dynamic to keep its shifting equilibrium in balance. Healing is the establishment of a new dynamic, a new equilibrium. Death is the collapse of both. . . . The entire process is and will always be a mystery, in a cosmos unheeding of us.*

I might have added that death is the final equilibrium, the motionless one. Whatever was the prime mover in life, moves no more.

Since "equilibrium" has too much smell of stasis, my diary entry stressed the element of "dynamism." The organism needs both change and stability. When it experiences too sharp change, whether in itself or its environments, it gets thrown into disorder. It needs to reorient itself, establish a new pattern of order, before it experiences further change within that pattern.

Thus we move through the phases of the life journey, through crises and traumas to renewals. Severe illnesses, whether physical or mental, are of course the critical traumas. Even if they don't assume terminal form, they throw us into disorder, threatening our life patterns.

I add a later journal note from August 1987, headed "Re order and disorder in a metaphysic of healing":

The thing we feel most in grave illness is the disorder. *We lose our center of gravity. Our physiological body image gets distorted. Our whole being yearns toward restoring order. Hence the importance that our rituals of order assume, not only in sickness but in healing. I have in mind the rituals of sleep and waking, of work and play, of punctual medication, of the orderly patterns of the day which we are more likely to strive for in sickness—and in healing—than in unthinking health.* (pp. 48–52)

DOWN BUT NOT OUT

EILEEN SHARP is a staff nurse on the hospice unit at the VA Medical Center in Wilkes-Barre, Pennsylvania. She wrote about her experiences "from the other side of the sheets."

Although I've been a nurse for many years, I never really appreciated my profession until I went through a life-threatening illness. Nor did I have any real idea of what it's like to be a patient until I became one.

Recovering from a bout of flu, I'd felt weak and lightheaded at work all day. That evening at the hairdresser's the room began to spin, and I felt myself slide out of the chair and onto the floor. Though I appeared unconscious and couldn't speak or open my eyes, I could hear and understand everything. I heard the hairdresser frantically call the police and my family. As the ambulance sped to the hospital, I heard an attendant say I had no blood pressure.

"Start a line," a voice said as I was wheeled into the ED. "This bitch has no veins," another voice complained. Ill as I was, I wondered how many patients like me hear remarks they shouldn't.

Finally they started a line and began infusing dopamine. I was able to open my eyes. But every time they tried to reduce the dose, I passed out again.

How strange it was to experience the hospital from a bed, hooked up to four IVs, a cardiac monitor, O_2, and a Foley catheter. Because of my low blood pressure I felt terribly cold. I asked for six or seven blankets and to be moved to a warmer spot on the unit. How many times had I wondered how a patient could want so many blankets, when I was perfectly warm. Now I understood.

I was besieged with specialists asking the same questions over and over, trying to discover the reason for my condition. I became grimly aware of how tiring such questioning is.

I was sent, without explanation, for X-rays and lung scans. I remembered sending my patients to undergo similar tests and not giving a thought to the apprehension that they might have been feeling.

I had severe nausea and vomited frequently. Once I began vomiting right after my morning care. Since both my hands were taped to IV boards, I could not reach the emesis basin. How easy it is, I remembered, to move things out of our patients' reach without realizing we have done it. Yet, somehow, it is the patient who winds up feeling guilty—for needing to be cleaned up again.

Things got worse before they got better. As the IVs kept infusing, I became more and more congested, with moist respirations and a persistent, productive cough. Another X-ray confirmed severe pulmonary edema from fluid overload. IV furosemide (Lasix) burned as it was injected. I'd given the drug many times without knowing it could cause such a sensation.

I learned, as well, how exhausted a very sick person feels. A 10-minute visit from a member of my family, or even a simple task—like trying to feed myself some Jell-O—left me completely drained.

Throughout this ordeal I had one emotional anchor: the night nurse. She spent so much time with me I doubt her care plans were up to par. But what a comfort she was! She made me tea to help control my nausea and rubbed my back when I was uncomfortable from trying to lie still amidst all the tubing. Each night I looked forward to her arrival, and I felt more secure with her around. I began to understand how the simplest acts can make a patient feel so much more cared for.

Eventually my blood pressure held when they tapered the dopamine. I was transferred to a med/surg unit. Sitting in a wheelchair, still hooked up to my IVs, catheter, and telemetry, I realized how these appendages impede normal movement. Is it any wonder that some of our patients move so slowly, when we are in such a hurry?

It took me several months to recover fully. They never found out what was wrong with me. My cardiologist speculated that the flu virus might have attacked the heart muscle and brain, resulting in a kind of viral myocarditis. The hospital report, though, said, "etiology unknown."

But even though I'll never know what hit me, I do know that I'm a different nurse because of it. Now I work on a hospice unit. Remembering how I could hear even when apparently unconscious, I encourage relatives to tell dying family members how much they love them. Knowing how tiring it is to be stuck with needles all the time, I empathize with patients who've had chemotherapy. Being aware how monumental the simplest task seems to a very sick patient, I give all the help and encouragement I can. I treat each patient as I would want to be cared for. (pp. 27–28)

Pain and suffering have their own literature, as is illustrated in the three selections below.

THE MYSTERY OF PAIN

EMILY DICKINSON

> Pain has an element of blank;
> It cannot recollect
> When it began, or if there were
> A day when it was not.
>
> It has no future but itself,
> Its infinite realms contain
> Its past, enlightened to perceive
> New periods of pain. (p. 10)

FLASHBACKS: THE CHARACTER OF PAIN

M. KELLY SIEVERS, a nurse anesthetist from Oregon, reached out to her peers through the Reflections column of the American Journal of Nursing *in 1989.*

I'd had major surgery for the first time, an abdominal hysterectomy. I am a nurse, yet I had no idea how the pain might claim me. After surgery, I lay awake flashing back over 25 years of nursing.

The scene is the shiny vinyl lobby of a small hospital. I'm a candy striper eagerly sitting at the front desk. I'm taken aback by a man rushing in, his hand dripping blood through a towel. I hear the nun telling him we can't help him. She directs him to a hospital with an emergency room. I mop the man's blood from green linoleum, and resume directing visitors to patients' rooms.

Pain aborts the drama. Like the man I, too, was cut. But I feel no knife-like sharpness. My pain is like a fist penetrating deeper and deeper into my abdomen. Despite the pillows that brace me, front and back, it is pain that holds me, that freezes my position. Hoping to fare better than the man who found no help, I call for a nurse and drift back to another of my memory's set stages.

The scene opens on a long wing of a large medical center. My 20-year-old self tells a postop patient it's too soon for more pain medicine. I suggest a change of position, but she clenches the side rail, unable to move. "If I hurt, why can't I have it?" She cannot argue when I reply, "You don't want to become addicted, do you?"

Later, I'm called into the instructor's office and told never to threaten a patient with drug addiction. But no one tells me what my lines should have been. We never reshoot the scene.

A nurse answers my call light. Today (my third day postop), I'd progressed to PO analgesics. But now it's 2 AM and I can't move or sleep. I want real relief, a shot of meperidine (Demerol).

The nurse is defensive—not because I'll become a drug addict, but because the rules of early discharge warn that a step back to IM analgesics might mean another day in the hospital. Patients don't take IM Demerol home with them.

"You took oral pain medicine today. Why not try it now?" she suggests. Everyone knows oral Demerol doesn't work, but I give in. I recycle the drug's euphoria down deep into my psyche, to wherever endorphins reside. The pressure lifts and my early nursing performances resume.

I'm 28 now, three months into anesthesia training. My instructor tells me to give the patient "what she needs." I'm still dependent on formulas and figures, which tell me she's had enough. I protest, but my instructor tells me again to give her what she needs.

A few more days bring new varieties of pain—shooting gas pains, punishing bladder spasms, and agonizing constipation. Incisional pain gnaws at me as I shuffle along the hallways. But the nurses on this set know the right lines. They follow the old maxim and give me what I need. I start to heal, unaware that another form of pain lurks just around the bend.

I'm in a pediatric ICU in a hospital well known for cardiac surgery. I'm 20 and feeding an infant who has an inoperable heart defect. For him, breathing is labor, eating is a task, and being fed is an assault. He cries, coughs, and turns blue. I have no lines. As I wait for him to recover, I see his mother crying at the window. She has not been able to visit him the last few days. She knows he will die. If I knew the right lines, I'd rush out to comfort her.

I'm going home tomorrow. I feel human again. I chat with a nurse as she lingers, making my bed. She explores my feelings of loss related to having a hysterectomy.

"I dealt with that last year when I had my tubal ligation," I assure the nurse. "I made a firm decision not to have children."

"Just don't be surprised if you find yourself having to deal with your feelings all over again," she cautions. I reflect on the courage and caring she has shown by treading onto my personal ground.

Baskets of flowers, cards, stuffed animals, and good wishes set the stage for my discharge. Suddenly, I become acutely aware of how my exit from the hospital mimics that of so many new mothers. A new pain appears: an aching jolt as I realize I'll never leave the hospital with a newborn infant of my own.

"Ready to go?" my nurse asks, and I remember my first night's fears. Pain. I really didn't know how its grip would claim me. (p. 784)

SUFFERING

RAM DASS, a.k.a. Richard Alpert, has taught at Harvard, Stanford, and the University of California. During his study of consciousness in India, he was given the name Ram Dass (Servant of God) by his guru, Neem Karoli Baba. PAUL GORMAN has taught at Sarah Lawrence College, City University of New York, Adelphi University, the Naropa Institute, and the Omega Institute. The following excerpt is from their book, How Can I Help?

Suffering seems to be a fact of life. How do we face it? Clearly it is a stranger to none of us. Perhaps we've not experienced the corrosive pain of illness, persecution, starvation, or violence. We may not have lived with the deterioration and loss of a loved one. Few of us have seen the charred face of a burned child. But each of us has experienced our fair share of not getting what we want or having to deal with what we don't want. In this, we all know suffering.

The way in which we deal with suffering has much to do with the way in which we are able to be of service to others. Of course, not all helping revolves around suffering. Much of what we offer may be in the nature of simple support or guidance: moving a friend's new furniture, teaching a child to read. But it is the affliction of others that most directly awakens in us the desire to be of care and comfort.

The impulse to do all we can to relieve one another's pain is the automatic response of our native compassion. But the experience of suffering—in ourselves and in others—triggers off complicated reactions. To investigate these is itself an act of compassion, an essential step toward becoming more effective instruments of mutual support and healing. How then do we respond to the pain we see around us? And, once we have investigated this response, how do we respond to our own afflictions? . . . (pp. 54–55)

Fear is the mind's reaction against the inherent generosity of the heart. Because the heart knows no bounds to its giving, the mind feels called upon to define limits. Under such tension, little wonder our choices of how to respond to the pain of others seem so difficult. . . . (p. 58)

Perhaps the strategy for dealing with suffering most familiar in our helping institutions is that of "professional warmth." Like pity, it's a stance to keep our distance. Since many professionals even believe that it's appropriate "not to get involved," they demonstrate a cool efficiency and impersonal friendliness, at best a façade, at worst plain hypocrisy. They become like their machines: cool green, giving off a competent hum. It's a way of plasticizing human relationships to keep them sterile, free of contact germs.

Of course it's understandable how this state of affairs has evolved. The demands on helping professionals to confront so much suffering each day are immense. "Professional warmth" is a survival strategy. But it's no answer. Our hearts pay the price, helpers and helped alike. . . . (pp. 62–63)

Denial, abstraction, pity, professional warmth, compulsive hyperactivity: these are a few of the ways in which the mind reacts to suffering and attempts to restrict or direct the natural compassion of the heart. This tension between head and heart leaves us tentative and confused. As we reach out, then pull back, love and fear are pitted against one another. As hard as this is for *us,* what must it be like for those who need our help? . . . (p. 64)

So we have to find tranquillity even in the midst of trauma. What's required is to cultivate a dispassionate Witness within. This Witness, as it grows stronger, can see precisely how we jump the gun in the presence of pain. It notices how our reactions might be perpetuating denial or fear or tension in the situation, the very qualities we'd like to help alleviate. The Witness catches us in the act, but gently, without reproach, so we can simply acknowledge our reactivity and begin to let it fall away, allowing our natural compassion to come more into play. The Witness gives us a little room.

Not only does it notice our own reactivity, but it also brings into the light of awareness the actions and reactions of other parties in the situation. Now we can begin, perhaps for the first time, to hear *them*. Less busy pushing away suffering, less frenzied having to do something about it, we're able to get a sense of what *they're* feeling, of what *they* feel they need. We may be startled to discover that what they've been asking for all along is entirely different from what we've been so busy offering: "All I want is for you to sit down here next to me. I don't care about the nurse; the IV is working fine; the bed is comfortable. Just sit with me." Quieter now, we can recognize such a need—often without it having to be expressed, perhaps even before it's consciously felt. We'll just come into the room and sit down and say "Hello."

This process of witnessing is dispassionate. It's not committed to one result or another; it's open to everything. Because it has, so to speak, no ax to grind, it is more able to see truth. As the Tao Te Ching says, "The truth waits for eyes unclouded by longing."

The Witness, however, is not passive, complacent, or indifferent. Indeed, while it's not attached to a particular outcome, its presence turns out to bring about change. As we bring *what is* into the light of clear awareness, we begin to see that the universe is providing us with abundant clues as to the nature of the suffering before us, what is being asked, what fears have been inhibiting us, and, finally, *what might really help*. All we have to do is listen—really listen.

Such investigation and inquiry into *what is* infuses a situation with a quality of freshness and possibility. As we see how reactive we have been, we find ourselves opening to new responses. It was our own reactivity unacknowledged that cut off the spontaneity of our helping heart. Once it is acknowledged, however—and once we begin to work with it—a whole new level of creativity becomes possible. (pp. 67–69)

> The experience of living (and dying) with the ill has been described with a sense of sharing, of community, of compassion and mutual support.

THE LINE

SHARON OLDS, contemporary American poet, published her first collection of poems, Satan Says, *in 1980. She has received a National Endowment for the Arts grant and a Guggenheim Foundation Fellowship.* The Dead and the Living *(1983), from which this excerpt comes, won the 1984 National Book Critics' Circle Award for Poetry.*

When we understood it might be cancer,
I lay down beside you in the night,
my palm resting in the groove of your chest,
the rachis of a leaf. There was not question of
making love: deep inside my body that
small hard lump. In the half-light
of my half-life, my hand in the beautiful
sharp cleft of your chest, the valley of the
shadow of death,
there was only the present moment, and as you
slept in the quiet, I watched you as one watches
a newborn child, aware each moment of the
miracle, the line that has been crossed
out of the darkness. (p. 54)

THE OTHER SIDE OF ALZHEIMER'S

DOROTHY STONEMAN wrote this article that appeared in the January 1986 issue of Present Time *and was reprinted in 1992 by* Health *magazine.*

My mother was diagnosed as having Alzheimer's disease four years ago. My husband and daughter and I have just moved into her house to take care of her. Whenever I tell anybody about it, they commiserate with great feeling. "I know how terrible it must be for you, I am so sorry! Alzheimer's is such a terrible thing to have to live with!"

I'd like to tell about my mother from a completely different point of view.

My mother is in no physical pain. She is still quite self-sufficient physically. She gets up in the morning, takes a shower, dresses herself, washes out her underpants and her pantyhose, combs her hair, and comes downstairs to eat breakfast. It might be peas, or lettuce, or turkey soup, or mayonnaise. Whatever it is, it gets milk put on top of it. After breakfast she struggles to make a list of food for us to buy. Since she doesn't remember the names of any of the foods, she systematically takes items out of the refrigerator or out of the cupboard, and copies down the name of them on her little slip of paper. After about 40 minutes of painstaking and laborious research, she produces a list of five items, usually including milk, tuna fish, and cookies. She gets one of us to drive her to the store, where we help her to select the items, bring them home, and put them away. After that, she often goes back to bed. When she wakes up, she starts over again. She comes down to breakfast again and eats something else with milk on it.

Two years ago, she went with my husband and me to watch people play tennis. As they stepped onto the court she said, "Oh, are we going to do this?" I realized that she would be willing to try to play tennis. I went home quickly to get her sneakers. Sure enough, she donned the sneakers, took the tennis racket, stepped out on the court, and prepared to play tennis. She had on a dress and stockings, and it was high noon on a hot summer day. She is 73 years old and had not played tennis in 30 years. I lobbed the ball over the net to her, and sure enough, *whack,* she slapped it back across the net. Back and forth, back and forth, and she never missed the ball. My husband and I were agog. She, on the other hand, seemed to think it was quite an ordinary occurrence. After 40 minutes of tennis, she said she'd had enough.

On the way to the car, she said, "We should have started that sooner. That was fun."

This event gave us a clue to many subsequent days of pleasure. We took her canoeing. We took her to play Ping-Pong. We took her out to play baseball with a plastic bat and a whiffle ball. She was completely successful at each of these activities. To find that my mother, who could no longer speak in coherent sentences, could actually play croquet, tennis, and Ping-Pong better than my ten-year-old daughter was amazing.

Two years ago she unexpectedly sat down at the piano, which she hadn't touched in 20 years, took out a Christmas music book and began to sight-read Christmas carols. She was most critical of herself, expressing disappointment at each note that she missed. We were amazed. She could no longer read English, yet she could sight-read music after not having done it for 20 years.

For my mother, Alzheimer's is not the worst way to die. At least she's always in a good humor, smiling lovingly at the people around her, saying, "Oh, I'm so glad to see you." "Very good!" "Oh, really!" "Oh, I'm so glad you came to my place!" Perhaps most important, she is surrounded by her family, who love her dearly. Without Alzheimer's she would not have been surrounded by her family, because she has always been completely self-contained and self-sufficient, encouraging independence among all her children. Had she died like her mother, with a quick heart attack when nobody expected it, none of us would have had the chance to express how deeply and how much we love her. This long, slow dying process of Alzheimer's has allowed each of us, in turn, to move in with her, to care for her, to give her everything she gave us as children. It is already six months to a year since she recognized any of us. Nonetheless, we know that she is she. We love her very much. (pp. 86, 88–89)

THE PARABLE

ROBERT M. WACHTER is a San Francisco physician, and the author of The Fragile Coalition: Scientists, Activists and AIDS, *in which the following parable serves as prologue.*

God and a rabbi are discussing heaven and hell. "I will show you hell," said God, and they went into a room that had a large pot of stew in the middle. The smell was delicious, but around the pot sat people who were famished and desperate. All were holding spoons with very long handles that reached to the pot, but because the handles of the spoons were longer than their arms, it was impossible to get the stew back in their mouths. Their suffering was terrible.

"Now I will show you heaven," said God, and they went into an identical room. There was a similar pot of stew, and the people had identical spoons, but in this room they were well-nourished and happy, talking with each other.

At first the rabbi did not understand. "It is simple," said God. "You see, these people have learned to feed each other."

TO THE WIFE OF A SICK FRIEND

EDNA ST. VINCENT MILLAY (1853–1950) wrote and published her poetry for nearly four decades. A graduate of Vassar College, she won the Pulitzer Prize for poetry in 1923 with The Harp Weaver.

Shelter this candle from the wind.
Hold it steady. In its light
The cave wherein we wander lost
Glitters with frosty stalactite,
Blossoms with mineral rose and lotus,
Sparkles with crystal moon and star,
Till a man would rather be lost than found:
We have forgotten where we are.

Shelter this candle. Shrewdly blowing
Down the cave from a secret door
Enters our only foe, the wind.
Hold it steady. Lest we stand,
Each in a sudden, separate dark,
The hot wax spattered upon your hand,

The smoking wick in my nostrils strong,
The inner eyelid red and green
For a moment yet with moons and roses,—
Then the unmitigated dark.

Alone, alone, in a terrible place,
In utter dark without a face,
With only the dripping of the water on the stone,
And the sound of your tears, and the taste of my own.

(pp. 209–210)

And the ill have appealed to the healer to be seen as a whole person, or, failing that, just as a person.

How Can I Help?

Ram Dass and Paul Gorman

I've been chronically ill for twelve years. Stroke. Paralysis. That's what I'm dealing with now. I've gone to rehab program after rehab program. I may be one of the most rehabilitated people on the face of the earth. I should be President.

I've worked with a lot of people, and I've seen many types and attitudes. People try very hard to help me do my best on my own. They understand the importance of that self-sufficiency, and so do I. They're positive and optimistic. I admire them for their perseverance. My body is broken, but they still work very hard with it. They're very dedicated. I have nothing but respect for them.

But I must say this: *I have never, ever, met someone who sees me as whole. . . .*

Can you understand this? Can you? No one sees me and helps me see myself as being complete, as is. No one really sees how that's true, at the deepest level. Everything else is Band-Aids, you know.

Now I understand that this is what I've got to see for myself, my own wholeness. But when you're talking about what really hurts, and about what I'm really not getting from those who're trying to help me . . . that's it: that feeling of not being seen as whole. (pp. 27–28)

THE BODY AS TERRITORY

ARTHUR FRANK is the author of numerous scholarly articles in medical sociology; he lives in Calgary, Alberta. At the Will of the Body (1991) was written following his experience with two major illnesses: heart attack and cancer.

The night before I had surgery, I was visited by an anesthesiologist who represented the culmination of my annoyance with . . . nonrecognition. He refused to look at me, and he even had the facts of the planned operation wrong. When he was leaving I did the worst thing to him I could think of: I made him shake hands. A hand held out to be shaken cannot be refused without direct insult, but to shake a hand is to acknowledge the other as an equal. The anesthesiologist trembled visibly as he brushed his hand over mine, and I allowed myself to enjoy his discomfort. But that was only a token of what I really wanted. I wanted him to recognize that the operation I was having and the disease it was part of were no small thing.

The kind of recognition I wanted changed over the course of my illness. While seeking diagnosis I felt that I was in a struggle just to get physicians to recognize the disease; once I got them onto the stage of my illness, the problem was to keep it my drama, not theirs. The active roles in the drama of illness all go to physicians. Being a patient means, quite literally, being patient. Daily life in the hospital is spent waiting for physicians. Hospitals are organized so that physicians can see a maximum number of patients, which means patients spend maximum time waiting. You have to be patient. Maybe the doctor will come this morning; if not, maybe this afternoon. Decisions about treatment are stalled until the doctor's arrival; nurses and residents don't know what's happening. Hopes, fears, and uncertainty mount.

When the physician does arrive, he commands center stage. I write "he" because this performance is so stereotypically masculine, although women physicians learn to play it well enough. The patient hangs on what brief words are said, what parts of the body are examined or left unattended. When the physician has gone, the patient recounts to visitors everything he did and said, and together they repeatedly consider and interpret his visit. The patient wonders what the physician meant by this joke or that frown. In hospitals, where the patient is constantly reminded of how little he knows, the physician is assumed not only to know all but to know more than he says.

In becoming a patient—being colonized as medical territory and becoming a spectator to your own drama—you lose yourself. First you may find that the lab results rather than your body's responses are determining how you feel. Then, in the rush to treatment, you may lose your capacity to make choices, to decide how you want your body to be used. Finally, in the blandness of the medical setting, in its routines and their discipline, you may forget your tastes and preferences. Life turns to beige. It is difficult to accept the realities of what physicians can do for you without subordinating yourself to their power. The power is real, but it need not be total. You can find places for yourself in the cracks.

I want to affirm the importance, both for yourself and for those around you, of holding onto the person you still are, even as medicine tries to colonize your body. Disease cannot be separated from other parts of a person's identity and life. Disease changed my life as husband, father, professor, and everything else. I had to learn to be dependent. I was unreliable in practical matters and often in emotional ones as well, and incapable of doing tasks that I had considered normal. It was no small thing to rediscover myself as I changed.

I have learned that the changes that begin during illness do not end when treatment stops. Life after critical illness does not go back to where it was before. A danger of allowing physicians to dominate the drama of illness is that they leave as soon as the disease is resolved to their satisfaction or when they have done all they can. Then the ill person and those around him are left to deal with the consequences of what has not been recognized. If the ill person dies, those who survive must deal with all that was not said, the unfinished business of a life closed out in a setting where dying is a problem of management, not a continuity of experience. And those ill persons who recover must recover not only from the disease but from being a patient. This recovery will proceed far more smoothly if the person within the patient has been recognized throughout the period of illness and recovery.

Continuing to recognize myself as the person undergoing the illness, reclaiming my body as my territory while I was in settings dominated by what was relevant to medicine alone, was no easy business. (pp. 55–58)

> In a later segment, Frank implores health professionals to recognize that they share the illness and support the ill.

To live among others is to make deals. We have to decide what support we need and what we must give others to get that support. Then we make our "best deal" of behavior to get what we need. This process is rarely a conscious one. It develops over a long time in so many experiences that it becomes the way we are, or what we call our personality. But behind much of what we call personality, deals are being made. In a crisis such as illness the terms of the deal rise to the surface and can be seen more clearly.

One incident can stand for all the deals I made during treatment. During my chemotherapy I had to spend three-day periods as an inpatient, receiving continuous drugs. In the three weeks or so between treatments I was examined weekly in the day-care part of the cancer center. Day care is a large room filled with easy chairs where patients sit while they are given briefer intravenous chemotherapy than mine. There are also beds, closely spaced with curtains between. Everyone can see everyone else and hear most of what is being said. Hospitals, however, depend on a myth of privacy. As soon as a curtain is pulled, that space is defined as private, and the patient is expected to answer all questions, no matter how intimate. The first time we went to day care, a young nurse interviewed Cathie and me to assess our "psychosocial" needs. In the middle of this medical bus station she began asking some reasonable questions. Were we experiencing difficulties at work because of my illness? Were we having any problems with our families? Were we getting support from them? These questions were precisely what a caregiver should ask. The problem was where they were being asked.

Our response to most of these questions was to lie. Without even looking at each other, we both understood that whatever problems we were having, we were not going to talk about them there. Why? To figure out our best deal, we had to assess the kind of support we thought we could get in that setting from that nurse. Nothing she did convinced us that what she could offer was equal to what we would risk by telling her the truth.

Admitting that you have problems makes you vulnerable, but it is also the only way to get help. Throughout my illness Cathie and I constantly weighed our need for help against the risk involved in making ourselves vulnerable. If we did not feel that support was forthcoming, we suppressed our need for expression. If we had expressed our problems and emotions in that very public setting, we would have been extremely vulnerable. If we had then received anything less than total support, it would have been devastating. The nurse showed no awareness or appreciation of how much her questions required us to risk, so we gave only a cheerful "no problems" response. That was all the setting seemed able to support.

Maybe we were wrong. Maybe the staff would have supported us if we had opened up our problems with others' responses to my illness, our stress trying to keep our jobs going, and our fears and doubts about treatment. We certainly were aware that our responses cut off that support. It was double or nothing; we chose safety. Ill persons face such choices constantly. We still believe we were right to keep quiet. If the staff had had real support to offer, they would have offered it in a setting that encouraged our response. When we were alone with nurses in an inpatient room, the questions they asked were those on medical history forms. In the privacy of that room the nurses were vulnerable to the emotions we might have expressed, so they asked no "psychosocial" questions.

It was a lot of work for us to answer the day-care nurse's questions with a smile. Giving her the impression that we felt all right was draining, and illness and its care had drained us both already. But expending our energies this way seemed our best deal.

Anyone who wants to be a caregiver, particularly a professional, must not only have real support to offer but must also learn to convince the ill person that this support is there. My defenses have never been stronger than they were when I was ill. I have never watched others more closely or been more guarded around them. I needed others more than I ever have, and I was also most vulnerable to them. The behavior I worked to let others see was my most conservative estimate of what I thought they would support.

Again I can give no formula, only questions. To the ill person: how much is the best deal costing you in terms of emotional work? What are you compromising of your own expression of illness in order to present those around you with the cheerful appearance they want? What do you fear will happen if you act otherwise? And to those around the ill person: What cues are you giving the ill person that tell her how you want her to act? In what way is her behavior a response to your own? Whose denial, whose needs?

Fear and depression are a part of life. In illness there are no "negative emotions," only experiences that have to be lived through. What is needed in these moments is not denial but recognition. The ill person's suffering should be affirmed, whether or not it can be treated. What I wanted when I was most ill was the response, "Yes, we see your pain; we accept your fear." I needed others to recognize not only that I was suffering, but also that we had this suffering in common. I can accept that doctors and nurses sometimes fail to provide the correct treatment. But I cannot accept it when medical staff, family, and friends fail to recognize that they are equal participants in the process of illness. Their actions shape the behavior of the ill person, and their bodies share the potential of illness.

Those who make cheerfulness and bravery the price they require for support deny their own humanity. They deny that to be human is to be mortal, to become ill and die. Ill persons need others to share in recognizing with them the frailty of the human body. When others join the ill person in this recognition, courage and cheer may be the result, not as an appearance to be worked at, but as a spontaneous expression of a common emotion. (pp. 68–71)

Note

1. Remen, Naomi (1980). *The human patient* (pp. 183–184). Garden City, NY: Anchor Press.

V

On Healing and Recovery

*C*atch hold of a peace deep within and push it into the
cells of the body.
With the peace will come back the health.

The Mother, *Seeds of Light*

The healing process continues to fascinate and often mystify
the healers as well as the healed. And the awesome nature of healing has inspired many writers. These selections on healing and
recovery range broadly from the philosophical, political, and personal to the poetic.

* * *

The Healing for Which We Took Birth

*Stephen Levine, a poet, teacher of meditation, and former editor
of the* San Francisco Oracle, *is a co-author of* Grist for the Mill
and has been a director of the Hanuman Foundation Dying

Project. He is widely known for his work with those con-
fronting death and grief. His book, Who Dies?, *is often used by*
hospices and universities as a teaching text. This selection ap-
peared in Healers on Healing, *1989.*

One way to approach the essential elements in healing is from the standpoint of the suffering we all share, the place we feel un-healed. What we regard as suffering or as unhealed is partially a question of perception, because much of what we call unhealed is that to which we have resistance, such as pain.

Suppose you stub your toe. What kinds of energy have you been conditioned to send into that throbbing discomfort? Most of us are taught to send fear and anger, even hatred, into our pain. Which, then is the unhealed—the throbbing toe or the hateful response to the unpleasant sensation?

Clearly, both factors are involved in our suffering. So true healing, which addresses the whole problem rather than partial manifesta-tions, always involves meeting suffering with loving-kindness, awareness, mercy, and balance, instead of trying to drive it away with fear, distrust, anger, and loathing.

If we look into the mind and heart, we see that no remedy is more radical or more natural than to meet hatred and fear with mercy and loving-kindness. Even in the cases of people who have used powerful medicines to meet powerful illnesses—for example, chemotherapy or radiation treatment for cancer—we have seen that the real healing seems to have been marked by the ability to relinquish the suffering, to let the healing in. Indeed, in our work with dying patients, we have observed many examples of those who hated their treatment so much, who encapsulated their ill-ness in such thick walls of resistance and fear, that it seemed a miracle if any of the chemotherapy or radiation could reach its target.

Healing, then, can be regarded as the establishment of a balance and equanimity in the midst of discomfort and agitation. We are healed when we can bring forth harmony out of the discordant strains of our life. And . . . one of the most effective ways of es-tablishing such a balance and harmony is through care.

. . . the word *care* is derived from the same root as *culture*. To bring oneself back into the common flow, the shared culture where the mind can relate to the body with heartfulness and mercy, is one of the bases of healing.

Another way of putting it is to say that an essential factor in all healing is love. For if the healer does not relate to that which calls out for healing with care, attention, and mercy—all aspects of love—then little healing can come about. Or, if there is "healing," it may be quite shallow, leaving the roots of the illness intact. Then the person "healed," although relieved of physical pain, remains with mental and spiritual pain untouched.

So many surface "healings" of this sort have left us unhealed. So many questions have been answered too quickly, thereby stopping the deeper investigation of the source of suffering in our lives. Often, it is discomfort in the body that puts us in touch with discomfort in the mind. To heal the body without including the mind, without allowing the body/mind to sink into the heart, is to continue the grief of a lifetime.

Another common denominator in the healing process is . . . grace. But grace is a word much misunderstood. It is not a power that comes from without, from above, from elsewhere. Grace is our true nature; it is the source of healing that we carry within us.

So the closer we come to our true nature, the closer we come to the healing for which we took birth. Many, indeed most, people never focus on that profound inner healing power that seeks to bring balance to the mind so that the heart can shine through beyond hindrance or obstruction. In fact, for many people it is not until they experience a physical illness that they become concerned with the great inner healing faculty.

Real healing never stops. It cannot, for it is our birthright, our essential nature. It is the continuing expansion of the "big bang" of birth, constantly creating universes to be explored and merged into. To discover this inner grace in each moment is to become healed. It is to discover the human divine within, the very source of healing, the essence of the deathless, the ever-healed.

Some years ago, I worked with a woman who was hospitalized with bone metastasis, cancer that had infiltrated the bone and resulted, in her words, in a "burning agony." Her lifestyle and her way of relating to the world were such that she had mercilessly judged all those with whom she had come in contact. She had been a tough businesswoman and a difficult parent—to such a degree that, although she was apparently dying of cancer, her children would not visit her, having been pushed out of her heart and out of her life so often.

This woman had never met her grandchildren. Each nurse, doctor, or visitor who came into her room was greeted with anger and profanity. So she was usually alone in her misery, wrapped in self-pity and blaming others for her torment.

One night after six weeks in the hospital, when her pain was enormous, when the walls of resistance she had built to keep life and death away had become so strained that they could not withstand a moment's more pressure, the dam burst and her pain broke through. Then, perhaps for the first moment in her life, she drew a breath into her pain—a single breath. She surrendered for a moment and allowed the suffering to move through her, not resisting it as though it came from outside or was another's fault, but giving herself to it as her own.

She said later that in that moment—when the turbulent waters of her lifelong resistance and suffering broke through and swept over her as she lay on her side with enormous pain in her back, hips, and legs—she experienced herself not as that woman in the hospital, but as an Eskimo woman dying in childbirth. A moment later, she said, she was a black-skinned Biafran woman nursing a starving child from a slack breast, dying of hunger and disease. The next moment, she was another woman, lying beside a river in that same fetal position, her back crushed by a rockfall, dying alone.

Image after image arose, which she described afterwards as feeling the suffering of "ten thousand people in pain." After that experience, which broke her heart and brought her back into contact with herself, she realized, "It wasn't *my* pain; it was *the* pain.

When it moved from 'my' pain to 'the' pain, it moved from the insufferable to the compassionate."

She had gone from the separate to the universal and had discovered that, when it is "my" pain, in this tiny mind and body, there is too little room for all that suffering. But when it is "the" pain, there is all the room in the world. Then the belly can remain soft, the heart can remain open, and our capacity to heal ourselves becomes the capacity to touch all the suffering in the world with mercy, loving-kindness, and a deeper sense of unity.

In the next six weeks, until she died, her room became the center of healing within the hospital. Many of the nurses spent their breaks there because it was the place where love was most radiant and evident. Within a week, after she had asked her children for forgiveness and pleaded for their return to her life, the grandchildren she had never met before were sitting next to her on the bed, playing "with Grandma . . . with Grandma's sweet, soft hands."

During those six weeks, the pain in her body diminished and the pain in her mind began to dissolve as her heart opened to encompass more and more life, more and more of that which is alive, and to touch the pain of all sentient beings with mercy and loving-kindness. We witnessed in that room one of the most remarkable healings we had ever seen. Although her body continued to deteriorate and she continued to be drawn gradually toward death, she died as healed as anyone we have ever seen. (pp. 196–199)

TRUST AND HONESTY: FOUNDATIONS OF HEALING

EMMETT E. MILLER is medical director of the Cancer Support and Education Center in Menlo Park, California. In addition to producing audio- and videotapes for self-healing and personal growth, he has authored Self-Imagery: Creating Your Own Good Health *and* Software for the Mind. *This is another selection from* Healers on Healing.

Two crucial requirements of the healing process are trust and honesty. By trust I mean that both the healer and the person to be healed have confidence that there is a power within the body that has the capacity to bring about healing when it is given the opportunity to do so. By honesty I mean the healer's willingness to be faithful and true to the spirit of the patient. . . . I have seen how both of these qualities must be present for any genuine healing to occur. They are key strands in the golden thread that binds together all methods of healing. (p. 119)

THE MYSTERIOUS PLACEBO

NORMAN COUSINS (1912–1990) was the author of twenty popular books including Anatomy of an Illness *and* The Healing Heart. *He served as the Editor of* Saturday Review of Literature *for many years, and later as chairman of the Task Force in Psychoneuroimmunology and adjunct professor of medical humanities in the School of Medicine at UCLA. The following is an excerpt from* Anatomy of an Illness, *1979.*

The placebo . . . is an emissary between the will to live and the body. But the emissary is expendable. If we can liberate ourselves from tangibles, we can connect hope and the will to live directly to the ability of the body to meet great threats and challenges. The mind can carry out its ultimate functions and powers over the body without the illusion of material intervention. "The mind," said John Milton, "is its own place, and in itself can make a heaven of hell, and a hell of heaven."

Science is concocting exotic terms like biofeedback to describe the control by the mind over the autonomic nervous system. But labels are unimportant; what is important is the knowledge that human beings are not locked into fixed limitations. The quest for perfectibility is not a presumption or a blasphemy but the highest manifestation of a great design.

Some years ago, I had an opportunity to observe African witchdoctor medicine at first hand in the Gabon jungle country. At the dinner table of the Schweitzer Hospital at Lambarene, I had ventured the remark that the local people were lucky to have access to the Schweitzer clinic instead of having to depend on witch-doctor supernaturalism. Dr. Schweitzer asked me how much I knew about witch doctors. I was trapped by my ignorance—and we both knew it. The next day *le grand docteur* took me to a nearby jungle clearing, where he introduced me to *un de mes collègues,* an elderly witch doctor. After a respectful exchange of greetings, Dr. Schweitzer suggested that his American friend be allowed to observe African medicine.

For the next two hours, we stood off to one side and watched the witch doctor at work. With some patients, the witch doctor merely put herbs in a brown paper bag and instructed the ill person in their use. With other patients, he gave no herbs but filled the air with incantations. A third category of patients he merely spoke to in a subdued voice and pointed to Dr. Schweitzer.

On our way back to the clinic, Dr. Schweitzer explained what had happened. The people who had assorted complaints that the witch doctor was able to diagnose readily were given special herbs to make into brews. Dr. Schweitzer guessed that most of those patients would improve very rapidly since they had only functional, rather than organic, disturbances. Therefore, the "medications" were not really a major factor. The second group had psychogenic ailments that were being treated with African psychotherapy. The third group had more substantial physical problems, such as massive hernias or extrauterine pregnancies or dislocated shoulders or tumorous conditions. Many of these problems required surgery, and the witch doctor was redirecting the patients to Dr. Schweitzer himself.

"Some of my steadiest customers are referred to me by witch doctors," Dr. Schweitzer said with only the slightest trace of a smile. "Don't expect me to be too critical of them."

When I asked Dr. Schweitzer how he accounted for the fact that anyone could possibly expect to become well after having been treated by a witch doctor, he said that I was asking him to divulge a secret that doctors have carried around inside them ever since Hippocrates.

"But I'll tell you anyway," he said, his face still illuminated by that half-smile. "The witch doctor succeeds for the same reason all the rest of us succeed. Each patient carries his own doctor inside him. They come to us not knowing that truth. We are at our best when we give the doctor who resides within each patient a chance to go to work."

The placebo is the doctor who resides within. (pp. 67–69)

Cousins has also described self-help and the "nourishing memory" in the following section of *The Healing Heart.*

BEYOND INVALIDISM

What can the individual do? First of all, it is important to be aware of the body's natural drive to heal itself, once freed of the provocations that played a part in bringing on the illness. If a person has a heart attack, for example, the first order of business is to attempt to perceive possible connections between that heart attack and the precipitating causes. If, as in my case, I was engaged in a losing war against congested highways, airport mazes, delayed checkins, overbooked planes, lost luggage, and late lecture arrivals, it was up to me to tame the schedule and make the necessary adjustments. Also, if my body craved exercise it was not receiving, only I was in a position to satisfy that want. And if my physical nourishment had to be augmented with nutrients for the mind, including joyous thoughts and experiences, I could not expect others to meet those needs for me.

Each individual presides over the totality of himself or herself. Assuming life is worth living—and the act of reaching out for medical help is proof positive that we think it is—it is imperative that we take on that part of the battle that is uniquely ours. It is a serious error to think of medical treatment as a total answer to all the problems of illness. In the end, the war against serious illness calls not only for expert medical attention but also for a summoning of values. Victory may not always be possible—if it were, we would all live forever—but it is sometimes within reach even in cases when the conventional wisdom holds the opposite.

It is in this sense that we retain control—recognizing the existence of resources represented by the healing system and the belief system that activates it. And the belief system is not just a collection of mechanical parts but a confluence of values and attitudes—hope, faith, confidence, purpose, will to live, and a capacity for joyous living.

Few of us will pass through this lifetime without the challenge of one or more serious illnesses. We need not feel angry or guilty when that illness occurs, nor is it reasonable to expect that recovery is always within easy reach. But we have the obligation to ourselves and those we love not to invite defeat by being defeatist.

If it is true that nothing is more striking about how the human body functions than its regenerative drive, it is also true that the regenerative drive works better under some circumstances than others. What we think, what we believe, what we eat, and what we do with our bodies are all involved in the circumstances of regeneration.

If it is important to avoid a sense of defeat, it is equally important to avoid a sense of guilt when progress or recovery may not be possible. Although we want to be able to mobilize all the resources inside us and make the fullest use of the resources outside us, there are times when disease cannot be reversed. We need not feel, at such times, that we have somehow failed, or that our faith and hope were insufficient to our requirements. Nor need we feel that personal adequacy or character is measured only by the ability to prevail.

The ultimate truth about life is that it is transient. We have a certain margin for the pursuit of our aims; we have powerful natural assets in the form of the will to live and a joyous response to life. These assets serve us well and help us to make the most out of ourselves; but they are not eternal elixirs. To feel despair or guilt because we may not always be successful in overcoming illness is to put ourselves above the basic laws of life.

We are not capable of banishing death. The final triumph is beyond us. But we are entitled to the fullest measure of help the world has to offer, just as those who are close to us are entitled to feel that we ourselves have offered the best within us. Death becomes tragic only when we have allowed things to die inside us that give meaning to life.

Even when the verdict is certain, we are not barred from the exercise of powers that rarely come into play at other times. I think of Hans Zinsser, the physician-philosopher, stricken with incurable illness, writing about the wide range of new perceptions that enabled him to sense and see things he had never sensed or seen before. His book *As I Remember Him* is a tribute not just to the man but to the uniqueness of human life.

"My mind is more alive and vivid than ever before," he wrote during his illness. ". . . My sensitivities are keener; my affections stronger. I seem for the first time to see the world in clear perspective. I love people more deeply and comprehensively. I seem to be just beginning to learn my business and see my work in its proper relationship to science as a whole. I seem to myself to have entered into a period of stronger feelings and saner understanding."

Zinsser made an important discovery about life—the way time can be transformed into energy. Time is the most important capital we own. We can lose great fortunes, and, if we are lucky, we may be able to regain them. But time is the only source of wealth which, once spent, can never be regained. There is only a finite amount of it for every person. "Ask me for anything," Napoleon is supposed to have said at the height of his power, "and I will be able to give it to you. Anything, that is, except time."

The way we choose to live and the depth of our feelings, our ability to love and be loved and to take in all the colors of the world around us—these determine the worth and true extent of whatever time we have. The clock keeps ticking away. Our job is to put as much meaning as possible into the intervals between the ticks. A minute can open out into a vast realm in which all our senses, finely attuned, can come into full and splendid play—or those same senses can be shut down, imparting nothing to our years except numbers.

What makes time so valuable is that it is convertible into nourishing memory. Memory is where the proof of life is stored. It offers material for stock-taking and provides clues about where our lives are going. Serious illness can be redemptive if it opens the sluices of vital memory, sharpens the focus, transforms the improbable into the possible, and imparts a quality of high art to the gift of time. (pp. 229–232)

> Jeanne Achterberg, in her book, *Woman as Healer,* has written forcefully about the contrasts, real and otherwise, within the cultural and gender dimensions of healing, as is illustrated in the following excerpts.

JEANNE ACHTERBERG

The Feminine Perspective and Merger of the Cultural Myth

What is the feminine voice, and if fully expressed, how might it affect society, in particular the institutions related to health? The concept of the feminine—and masculine—voice, myth, perspective, or principle (terms used interchangeably) is derived from several sources: Eastern philosophy, personality theories (especially Carl Jung's), research on cognitive styles of males and females, and long-held and widespread cultural mythologies. The typical traits associated with masculine and feminine are relatively—but by no means completely—consistent across time and culture.

The masculine and feminine are regarded as polarities that, together, comprise the whole of the process of being. Neither aspect of the polarity is complete in and of itself; each depends upon the manifestation of its opposite for full expression. Men, of course, have a feminine aspect, and women, a masculine aspect. The myths no doubt have some basis in genetic differences but also are formed through environmental forces. . . . (pp. 190–191)

The Healer and the Healing System

In a balanced viewpoint that includes both the masculine and feminine perspective, healing is seen not as technique, but as process. The healing system moves beyond its intense and limited concentration on molecular biology to the integrity of community, environment, and concerns for the spirit. The healer takes on new dimensions, with wisdom gained from superb professional training as well as from the depths of personal experience. . . .

In a balanced system, neither healing nor curing is something that one person *does* to another. Instead, both terms refer to internal processes, reflecting a more basic definition of health which implies harmony and wholeness. As such, physical health—or the molecular biology—may or may not be changed or relevant to wholeness. The end-points of being "healed" or "whole" are more a matter of personal opinion than the results of a urinalysis, or a psychological test, or anyone else's criterion of what constitutes "well." Furthermore, through the healing process, a person may be more whole, more harmonious, or more "well" than before, having gained strength and insight. Disease or suffering, in fact, may be regarded as critical events in the path toward personal transformation.

I believe that a balanced view of healing would also include the following concepts:

1. Healing is a lifelong journey toward wholeness.
2. Healing is remembering what has been forgotten about connection, and unity and interdependence among all things living and nonliving.
3. Healing is embracing what is most feared.
4. Healing is opening what has been closed, softening what has hardened into obstruction.
5. Healing is entering into the transcendent, timeless moment when one experiences the divine.
6. Healing is creativity and passion and love.

7. Healing is seeking and expressing self in its fullness, its light and shadow, its male and female.

8. Healing is learning to trust life. (pp. 193–194)

And how does healing appear to the "wounded healer"? One such person, Max Lerner, illuminates the process in the passage that follows.

WRESTLING WITH THE ANGEL

MAX LERNER

During the ailing/healing years, I learned that the healing reality is not suspended in midair. Along with the network of neural receptors and messengers it has as base a spiritual reality which is grounded in survival but reaches to belief of some sort. The nature of that belief varies with cultures and theologies: the fact of it is common to all, just as the shamanic tradition, which joins spirituality and belief with healing, is found in some form in almost every culture.

The historian of religions, Mircea Eliade, noted that the shaman had himself often suffered a deep illness and in combatting it had been drawn to healing others. A similar insight may be found in Carl Jung's archetype of the "wounded healer." The common theme is the creative force evoked by illness that has been noted in the lives of great thinkers, artists, political and religious leaders.

One thinks of Charles Darwin, with his intolerable headaches, charting the evolution of man; of Sigmund Freud, with his cancer of the palate, invoking the life force to counter the death principle; of Milton Erickson, paralyzed, using hypnosis to animate the frozen psyches of patients; of Stephen Hawking, totally immobilized, spinning hypotheses of unification theory for the cosmos; and on a political level, of Franklin Roosevelt, also strapped in a wheelchair, teaching a fearful nation to recover its energies and walk.

It was an image never far from my thoughts. Every patient, as Albert Schweitzer saw, carries a doctor, as healer, within himself. Everything connected with illness is a wounding experience. It is an inspiriting thing to think of both patient and "doctor within the patient" as part of the healing process, and to see both as using the healing to recover from their wounds. . . . (pp. 109–110)

———

I pause again for a backward look on my illness to ask what the path was that led out of the wilderness to a clearing of some sort. The working-through effect I have mentioned, how did it *work* for me?

An analogy may be useful. In tracing the evolution of life, cosmologists speak of a *food chain* linking the common fate of living things: when it broke at a critical point, its effects were felt all down the line. So the principle of connectedness applies to the total human organism.

A possible metaphor is that of a *sickness chain* which operates with some sort of domino effect, as a dysfunction in one system exerts an adverse impact on others closely connected. But if a sickness chain why not also a *healing chain,* in which the return to functioning in one system exerts a positive effect on the others?

The domino image, with its implied principle of momentum, comes to mind. Granted, this isn't some impersonal principle of physics we are dealing with but a living organism. Yet in that organism the test should be not only in what happens on the downward slope, which is apparent enough, but on the upward slope, which researchers are only now starting in earnest to probe.

Just as I felt a downward domino effect in the turmoil of my clouded phase, so I felt a positive domino effect in the elation of the upward arc of healing. When I stopped losing weight during my first cancer and started to gain without food forcing, I had the pleasure of curbing my mounting appetite by a somewhat rational regimen. My new-found energy took me outdoors in walks, wood gathering, and tasks around our grounds. This helped my digestion and made me sleep better, without nightmares. The energy I got from walking and sleeping in turn enabled me to work more productively. My concentration improved, words came to me more readily, my imagery grew more confident. The memory losses that accompany illness and aging seemed minimized. My web of relations became closer and stronger.

Every new advance built on the sequence of all previous ones. I seemed to be on a euphoric binge. My work became more playful; my play allowed more scope for the mysterious processes of work. I had always tried to break down fences between work and play. I now found it easier to keep the fences from forming. The reality for me was something very like a reversal effect. After the shock and anguish, the stress and pain, the anxiety and fear, the bottoming out and the slow ascent, I began to have the feeling of putting it all together.

It is hard to fix on the exact occasion when the will to live asserted itself with a confidence that brooked no self-doubts. It was not a one-time thing that sprang full blown. In my most troubled illness years, after a note on some long-range project, I would jot down a phrase in my journal: "I *must* live."

I can't recall when the "must" became "I *can* live," turning resolve into possibility. It was the wager phase, a time when I hung on Dick Silver's battlefield dispatches as he reported the results of the blood tests. I would sit in the examining room, writing, but actually waiting tensely, watching his face as he entered the room, to detect what the smile or frown augured. I was like the Victorian reader who bought each issue of the magazine to see whether Charles Dickens or Anthony Trollope would kill off a character or let him live. It was life-or-death by installments, only in this case it was my own life.

The turning point came at one visit to Silver when the nurturing cell count moved upward. So did my heart. I noted it in my journal that day, and added, "I didn't take the bus home. I walked." It was my way of celebrating. The good news gave me the right to walk despite my weakness, but the jubilant walk in turn did wonders for my mind and doubtless for my cell count.

I couldn't will my mood out of the blue because I couldn't get away with fooling myself. But I could use some nurturing event to build a mood without feeling foolish. That was how I used all my good news.

Not all of my healing course had calm waters to sail on. There were hopes, but also dashed hopes. There were signals of increasing energy and also setbacks. Dick Silver, with all his encouragements, was careful not to raise my hopes, lest the fall be steep. Yet the auguries continued favorable, and the time came when I reached a new phase in my conjugation of the verb "live." After moving from "I must" to "I can" I took the final step. "I *will* live" I told myself, and while the element of sheer resolve was still present in "will," it was fused with an element of confidence I had not dared earlier.

How and when did this feeling come? The episode was so minor that it appears an anticlimax rather than epiphany. It centered on the opposite bank of the East River, which runs past our apartment as it also runs past the hospital a half-mile farther downtown. I used to stand at the window of my hospital room, looking across the river at the cars, buses, people. I watched them with envy. I once had their vigor. I would not have it, I thought, for long. Back at home, still struggling with my first cancer, I looked out every day over the same river at scenes on the other bank, still with envy tinged with sadness.

Then one day much later, when my lung complications were starting to resolve, just about the time I decided to put away my memoir and return to my ongoing daily work, I noticed something. As I looked out at the opposite bank, at the river and the tugs, it came to me that I no longer was sad about them, nor did I envy the people I saw. Instead I felt elated. I was part of them and they of me, part of the same enterprise of life which flowed out of me into an indefinite future, as the river flowed. (pp. 90–94)

The experience of recovery has also been described by a number of writers—sometimes in celebration, or sometimes with hesitation, skepticism, and even disbelief.

CEREMONIES OF RECOVERY

ARTHUR FRANK

Recovery deserves a ceremony. Many aboriginal peoples have reentry rituals during which a person who has been stigmatized is purified. These rituals are a rebirth; afterward life can begin anew. Each of my critical illnesses ended with a medical event that could have been given a ritual value. But physicians, the high priests of our time, have let themselves be reduced to mere medical technicians. They act as if they are unaware of the power of their interventions to change the body's symbolic value. Both the patient and physician are thus deprived of the spiritual experience of illness. Because ritual self-awareness is excluded from the system, it takes longer to work out one's own terms of reentry.

The angiogram which showed that my heart problems were over had ritual potential, and I had the sense to value the sight of my own heart beating. But medicine reduced the angiogram to the end of an incident. I accepted, even embraced, this reduction and did not try to experience it as the beginning of a life that was now different. The angiogram only signaled the end of a breakdown; it was not an occasion for rebirth.

After the angiogram I could believe that the incident was over. There had been a virus, but now it was gone. I had no more heart problems, period. After cancer, however, I had no such belief. Cancer never disappears. I read recently about a young man whose cancer recurred after a thirteen-year remission. Medical science is just beginning to understand cancer's capacity to be present in the body but inactive for decades. Cancer creates the disturbing image of the body as a time bomb, genetically programmed to explode at some future time. I could be having a recurrence now and not yet know it, or I could live another forty years and die of something else. You are never cured of cancer; you can only live in remission.

My remission began several weeks after the third round of chemotherapy. The CAT scan showed that the tumors had shrunk, but the reduction was no longer considerable. The remaining masses on the X-rays were assumed to be scar tissue, which would never disappear entirely but would continue to reduce gradually. The chemotherapy was judged to have done what it could. My treatment could end.

My intravenous line provided its last valuable service as the occasion of a ceremony. After reporting the scan, the physician left Cathie and me in a treatment cubicle while he prepared another room for the surgical procedure of pulling out the line. Its installation changed our relationship by requiring each of our days to begin and end with a focus on cancer. The care of the line had tied Cathie to me and tied us both to cancer; these ties had brought nuisance and caring, fear and possibility. Because of the line's symbolism, as well as its problems, we had looked forward to its removal as the beginning of life after cancer. My own emotions were intensified by the physical drain of preparing for the scan. I had not eaten in about twenty-four hours and had had almost no sleep. My physical reserves and our emotional reserves were gone, so we started to cry, in a mixture of joy, relief, and just plain breakdown.

When a nurse came into the room and saw us crying, she looked totally confused. Suddenly a light bulb went on. "I guess this must be kind of a big moment for you," she said. She was a good nurse and had been mercifully quick and efficient at getting prescriptions to manage painful side effects, but for her suffering was a problem of management, not a crisis of spirit. Her perceptions were always on the surface of bodies. That moment was one of the few times she saw beyond the disease to the experience of illness. She talked happily of former patients returning to see her when their hair had grown back; chemotherapy sounded like a problem of grooming. When hair returns, all is forgotten. But when all is forgotten, nothing is learned. Her way of seeing missed the ritual, which is a passage through real and symbolic dangers in preparation for the opportunity of a life enhanced by that passage.

The line was pulled, the incision sewed up. Medicine, as ritual, inflicted another mark on my body, giving that body a value it did not have before. Ritual markings are not just stigmas; scarification during an initiation rite marks the person as having passed through some level of experience, entitling him to higher status as a result. Thus initiated, my body was mine again. Life could begin once more. Of course I knew life had never stopped. The nights listening to Bach, the afternoon light on the Chagall print, the moments of hope and fear shared with Cathie, the losses and frustrations had been anything but life stopping during cancer. It had only intensified. If the months from the ultrasound in September to the removal of the line in January seemed like a lifetime, it was because during this time everything counted. I could not afford to let anything slip by unobserved and unfelt.

My life had not stopped, but a great deal of it had been put on hold. Now I could begin to make plans again, to think of travel, to commit myself to projects at work. The process of reentry was not smooth. I now knew that the way I and others lived was a choice, and often not the best one. My consciousness remained suspended between the insulated world of illness and the "healthy" mainstream. This suspension expressed itself in my lack of tolerance for tension and disagreements. I continued to value much of the life of an ill person, even though I was no longer officially diseased.

I still needed time to myself. It was warm in Calgary that winter, and I took long walks on the hills overlooking the river. I chose the time for these walks so that I would come over the crest of the hill just as the afternoon sun shone directly on the water. Chemotherapy had deprived me of air and sun. I wanted to store up these elements against the possibility that I might be deprived of them again. In that sunlight on the river I began to heal.

I become less and less a person with cancer, but the continuing schedule of examinations, X-rays, and blood tests reminds me that I remain at greater risk than others. This risk diminishes over time but never disappears. Life remains a remission. But my sense of being a person with cancer is on the level of experience, not of medicine. I do not want to take recovery too far. Part of the fear of dying is realizing all that I have not done or have not done enough of. As long as life remains a recovery, I try to seize the life I someday want to have lived. The value of remaining a person with cancer is to keep asking the question: If I get sick again, what will I tell myself about the way I spent my time?

I am also reminded of cancer when I meet people I see infrequently. Some ask, guardedly, how my health is. Their concern recognizes that cancer is never "over" in the way a virus is over when it passes out of the body. Others greet me by pronouncing, "You're fine." Theirs is less a question than a statement. I hear their wish that cancer never happens, and if it has to happen, that it be put away. I have assumed a dual presence for people. My being here suggests that cancer is not always fatal, but that it does happen. Some see the survival in the foreground and the risk in the background; for others the risk dominates. On different days I myself emphasize different halves.

I am trying, in this third year after cancer, to be a little less afraid. Some days the world seems immensely fearful, a place where some germ cell is waiting to explode. Another of Paul Simon's memorable lyrics says, "Somebody could walk into this room/ And say your life is on fire." One day during a self-examination I felt something I had not felt in the two years since surgery. I panicked but made an appointment to see the same urologist who had originally diagnosed me. A few days after Cathie and I were again waiting in a treatment ward, listening to the other patients through the thin curtains. We sat there waiting for the urologist, who could walk into that room and say our lives were on fire. But it did not happen that time. Whatever it was I had noticed, he pronounced me normal. We left, less happy than dazed by the vision of what might have happened. This vision gives each day its value. Of course the condition of my life is no different from anyone else's, but I get these reminders, for which I am grateful.

The only real difference between people is not health or illness but the way each holds onto a sense of value in life. When I feel I have no time to walk out and watch the sunlight on the river, my recovery has gone too far. A little fear is all right. It is all right to know that in a month I could be lying in a hospital bed asking myself how I spent today. Holding onto that question—how did you spend today?—reminds me to feel and see and hear. It is too easy to become distracted. When the ordinary becomes frustrating, I have to remember those times when the ordinary was forbidden to me. When I was ill, all I wanted was to get back into the ordinary flux of activity. Now that I am back in the ordinary, I have to retain a sense of wonder at being here.

Like Job, I have had my goods restored to me. Secure in the knowledge that I am dust, I enjoy what I have. I even run again, not as far or as fast, but with greater pleasure. Long runs let my mind drift to whatever fantasy comes along. Some days that fantasy turns to my death, but not in sadness. I wonder what kind of death I would need, to feel I had lived well. What I tell myself changes; all that matters is staying at peace with my own mortality.

I want to keep running, but someday I will have to stop. I do not know what that day will be like. If I have recovered well but not too much, I will remember a poem I keep over my desk by the late Raymond Carver, called "Gravy." A man, an alcoholic, is about to die, but he changes his habits and lives for ten years. Then he gets a brain disease and again is dying. He tells his friends not to mourn:

> I've had ten years longer than I or anyone
> expected. Pure gravy. And don't you forget it.

I try not to.

When I become ill again, and someday I will, I hope it will not be the total break in my life, the radical discontinuity, that I experienced before. Health and illness are not so different. In the best moments of my illnesses I have been most whole. In the worst moments of my health I am sick. Where should I live? Health and illness, wellness and sickness perpetually alternate as foreground and background. Each exists only because of the other and can only alternate with its other. There is no rest in either word. In "health" there can only be fear of illness, and in "illness" there is only discontent at not being healthy. In recovery I seek not health

but a word that has no opposite, a word that just is, in itself.
When I seek the meaning of my recovery, the opportunity of illness, I call it gravy. (pp. 129–135)

RECOVERING

*MURIEL RUKEYSER (1913–1980), one of America's most distin-
guished poets, produced 14 volumes of poems during her half-
century career. Her work reflected her belief that the concerns
of poetry and the concerns of life are inextricable. The following poem is taken from* The Gates, *1976.*

Dream of the world
speaking to me.

The dream of the dead
acted out in me.

The fathers shouting
across their blue gulf.

A storm in each word,
an incomplete universe.

Lightning in brain,
slow-time recovery.

In the light of October
things emerge clear.

The force of looking
returns to my eyes.

Darkness arrives
splitting the mind open.

Something again
is beginning to be born.

A dance is
dancing me.

I wake in the dark. (pp. 57–58)

VI

ON CARE, CARING,
AND CAREGIVING

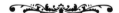

*C*are made a kind of family. When I walked through the dark streets to the subway to return home, I used to feel them all behind me, as if I were myself stretched out inside each one.

Anne Truitt, *The Journal of an Artist,* 1982

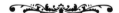

In the eternal quest for the meaning and significance of nursing, no word has been invoked so consistently as *care.* We have mined it as assiduously as prospectors searching for gold. In recent years, a whole literature has grown up around the concept. "Care" spans the ages, connecting nursing to its roots. It bridges the vocabulary of the nurse worker and the nurse theorist, sometimes gracefully, sometimes uneasily. It connects nursing to other "caring" professions and nurses to other "caregivers." It offers itself as the personal, yet shared frame of reference for the professional and the layperson. It is a concept for which we must have a clear and lasting affinity.

113

However, care and caring are so all-encompassing, connoting as they do both a state of mind (caring about) and a state of action (caring for), that they invite ambiguity and intellectual controversy. The crux of much of the controversy is the deceptive dichotomy between "emotional work" and "intellectual work" and the fear of being stigmatized as the former, depending upon the sway of social values. The term "caring" also fuels endless discourse about the difference between caring and curing and territorial claims to either or both.

The caring heart of nursing, as well as the heart of the caring debate, are the subjects of compelling literature. Although a small number of such pieces have been collected in this chapter, the concepts and the words pervade the book and form the matrix around which our profession is woven.

* * *

LETTERS TO OLGA

VACLAV HAVEL, dissident Czech poet and playwright, was blacklisted for his political activities by the Communist government, and his work prohibited from publication or performance after 1969. Letters to Olga, *written to his wife during his imprisonment, is excerpted here. He was elected President of Czechoslovakia in December 1989 after the fall of the Communist regime, and President of the Czech nation in 1993 after the partition of Czechoslovakia.*

Everything meaningful in life, though it may assume the most dramatic form of questioning and doubting, is distinguished by a certain transcendence of individual human existence—beyond the limits of mere "self-care"—toward other people, toward society, toward the world. Only by looking "outward," by caring for things that, in terms of pure survival, he needn't bother with at all, by constantly asking himself all sorts of questions, and by throwing himself over and over again into the tumult of the world, with the intention of making his voice count—only thus does one really become a person, a creator of the "order of the spirit," a being capable of a miracle: the re-creation of the world. To give up on any form of transcending oneself means, de facto, to give up on one's own human existence and to be contented with belonging to the animal kingdom.

The tragedy of modern man is not that he knows less and less about the meaning of his own life, but that it bothers him less and less. (p. 237)

> In *Composing a Life,* Bateson has devoted a valuable chapter to care and caregiving in relation to the self and to others.

CAREGIVING

MARY CATHERINE BATESON'S Composing a Life *is a study of her own life and the lives of four other women: Joan Erikson, author, dancer and teacher of dance, jewelry designer, and wife of Erik Erikson; Ellen Bassuk, physician and psychiatrist whose practice includes the homeless whose only health care is found in the emergency department of a Boston hospital; Alice d'Entremont, electrical engineer and CEO of a high-tech company in New England; and Johnnetta Cole, first African-American woman president of Spelman College in Atlanta, Georgia.*

How much care is needed and how much human effort needs to go into caretaking? There is no way to compute it, for the meaning of the word "care" is endlessly ambiguous: it has one meaning in a hotel and another in a hospital, one in a day-care center and another in a university. There are different needs for care between infants and adults, healthy and well, and great differences are made by training, skill, and equipment. Part of our blindness comes from the fact that in some situations, the need for care is urgent because of accident or earlier neglect; in others, invisible care routinely given has meant that no need is ever apparent. Any computation of dollars or numbers for such a spectrum is nonsense, but the image of the songbirds stands as a reminder that caretaking is essential to survival, while the connection between the number of eggs and the hours of daylight poses a question of the underlying mathematics of human caring. For human beings, "caring for" means far more than hunting for worms for a nestful of squawking fledglings; it emerges in every activity, from electrical engineering to bookkeeping to farming.

Today, we all risk being without needed care at some crucial moment, or of suffering from the effects on others of insufficient care. At one time, many men could assume that their wives would devote their lives to caring for them and their children; the elderly could once count on the care of their adult daughters and sons (or the sons' wives). Now, the problems of giving and receiving needed care force everyone to improvisation and patchwork. For all our elaboration of professional forms of caretaking, caretaking is necessarily dispersed through the society. It is a skill that everyone can usefully learn, practiced mutually, necessary both in the workplace and at home, and no longer attached to a fixed set of roles. When Joan and I were taping interviews, Erik developed a ritual of bringing us tea—caring for us but also soliciting care, checking in with Joan for reassurance about the plans of the day.

Homemaking can be done in tandem, but caretaking, even when two people alternate, is always a complementary relationship, never exactly symmetrical. One hopes that in a marriage the times of greatest need will not coincide, that when the one is most needy the other will find resources. But these rhythms of give and take are not easy to develop. Even at the dinner table, it takes skill to allow both partners enough of what my husband calls emotional air time to recite the troubles of the day and be comforted; it is harder still when the needs of the whole week must be compressed into a weekend. It can only work if each partner learns to find satisfaction in caring for the other, like learning to enjoy the mutual giving of pleasure in the syncopated rhythms of lovemaking.

We have also become increasingly thoughtful about the question of self-care. Some of this is fashion, some of it can be dismissed as narcissism or a new way of expressing affluence, but some of it is an investment in autonomy and in sustaining the quality of life through a longer maturity. We joke about women who urge their men, like children, to wear their galoshes or to get needed exercise, but it is a vast relief when these same men start to take some responsibility for their own well-being. Just as important, women need to care enough about themselves to care for themselves as more than the property of some man.

It is not easy to learn to cherish oneself when one's life has been organized around cherishing others or when all the cherishing has been delegated to someone else. During my Amherst years, on the weekdays of coming home to a single-parent household, I felt a weary envy of my predecessor, who had a full-time homemaker waiting for him. I justified the time I put into developing an exercise program or learning about computers by what these pleasures would enable me to offer the college. Still, I used to buy flowers and silk scarves as tokens of caring for myself and treat myself to long scented baths with the phone turned off. . . .

Today, those who begrudge themselves care, feeling that their role in life is to care for others, can be persuaded to think about issues of health and stress reduction. As a result, a little cherishing of the self is translated into responsible behavior, even a way of caring for others. . . . But self-care is important for its own sake as well. It is intimately tied to self-esteem, with the implication that the one who is cherished is important and valuable for his or her own sake.

Ellen has always moved between the issues of caretaking that accompany privilege and those that arise at the point of desperation. She was working as director of the psychiatric emergency service at Beth Israel Hospital when emergency wards, set up to deal with accidents and sudden emergencies, began to be flooded with patients with chronic complaints whose disrupted lives gave them no regular access to care. The appearance of the homeless on the streets of America is a visible reminder that while some Americans receive the most expensive and skilled forms of care, from organ transplants to psychoanalysis, others may be entirely alone and uncared for. The situation demands both new definitions of need and new institutions and highlights the fact that obtaining care is a skill. There is a necessary spectrum in which a commitment to care for the desperate balances the commitment to

provide intimate care within the household. Together, the two offer a perspective for creating a society adequately cared for. Every time we turn away from including compassion in the national
agenda, we handicap ourselves for real leadership. (pp. 142–146)

<hr />

Almost any activity can be interpreted at least in part as caretaking. One of the most striking aspects of the Eriksonian version
of the life cycle is that the basic strength that characterizes the
long adult years is the virtue of care. The achievements of maturity are described, for both men and women, in analogy with
parental responsibility, including the willingness to relinquish
control gradually and welcome the transition to an unknown future. At its best, care creates freedom. But even as almost any
activity can be informed by care, the caretaking professions
themselves can be distorted into forms of exploitation rather
than caring, with one asymmetrical relationship easily transmuted into another. Caring fathers and mothers can become
tyrannical patriarchs and matriarchs, devouring their children instead of nurturing them. Healing and helping can become forms
of domination, medical qualification an excuse for bullying. When
Ellen first talked to me about shelters, I was amused at the eu-
phemistic optimism of calling those driven to depend on them
"guests." After I began to get a sense of the pain and vulnerability
of the homeless, I began to see this terminology as a steady, careful reminder, against all evidence, of the value of respect and of
the freedom to move on.

It's a curious alchemy, the way caring enters into and transmutes
other activities. An interesting example is the Iditarod, the 1,157-
mile dogsled race across Alaska that has been won repeatedly by
a woman, Susan Butcher. This grueling course was first run to
save lives at a time when serum was desperately needed in Nome
to combat an epidemic. Now, as a race, the mode of caring and
service has been converted into competition, but it is clear that
even within the competitive framework, Butcher achieves excellence by conceptualizing the struggle in terms of caring for her

dogs. At every rest stop in the 1987 race, her rival Rick Swenson left early, while Butcher gave her dogs the full four-hour rest time; she was so busy caring for them that she had only fifteen minutes of rest for herself. By the end of each lap, her dogs were forging ahead of his. "My dogs just kept getting stronger and stronger," she told the *Boston Globe* (March 20, 1987). "They gained in power the further along we got." At the last rest stop, the rules of the race required Swenson to give his animals the full rest time. Butcher's lead became unbeatable. Where he was willing to overtax his dogs, she was willing to overtax herself, organizing her efforts around caring for her dogs. After the race, care for herself: a glass of wine, a hot bath, and sleep. It has been observed that in women's athletics, the women will stop playing when a teammate is injured, until she has been attended to, while male athletes will more quickly resume their competitive combat. Slowing down for caretaking is obviously a losing strategy in the short run, but a winning strategy in the long run, whether in a two-week race across Alaska or the life and survival of the human species on a planet that must be cherished, for it can never be replaced.

It is easy to think of caring in terms of embrace and nurture, in the image of a mother holding a child, but Ellen spoke of caring in terms of a quality of attention, a total commitment to looking and listening, that also reminded me of Vanni's infancy. "To do therapy," Ellen said, "you have to be unencumbered, so you can really listen reflectively and allow your free associations to be very present in your head and not be all cluttered with other things." This quality of attention has the same paradoxical quality as the need to be on duty twenty-four hours a day: it cannot be perfectly achieved, but it proposes the ideal that underlies real caring. No one is more attentive than a mother trying to learn to recognize and respond to the needs of a newborn. She sleeps, of course, but she is sensitive to cries even when she is busy or sleeping. There is a sense in which we need to turn that same kind of attention toward the fields we cultivate and the organizations we manage if these charges are to thrive.

Growing up with the capacity to care for people or communities or ideas depends on the early experience of receiving loving and effective care. It is the lack of this experience that turns home-lessness into a cross-generational disease. Caring can be learned, especially through the kind of total responsibility given to young doctors, but it requires a base of empathy built before internship or residency. Ellen sometimes found this base simply lacking. "It was my contention that you don't need to know a lot to work in the ER but you had to have some intuitive sense of how to take care of someone—that was always one of my hobby horses. In the ER you're at risk because they discharge people. Sometimes someone is discharged who is dangerous, really psychotic, and you wonder how the resident could possibly have missed it. Sometimes you have to follow a patient or hold their hand, and there are some people you just can't let walk out of there because you just know they are going right down the tubes. Some residents were fabulous caretakers and you never had to say another word, but some, no matter what you told them, they didn't have the foggiest idea about taking care of an ER patient. All you really needed to know was if somebody was in trouble. The rest was gobbledygook. Well, that's too reductionist, but there's an element of truth in that. I actually gave some residents a hard time around their inability to take care of people. The bottom line is that there are people who are good caretakers and some that you wouldn't want taking care of your horse."

Today there are many people who decide not to have children, but this decision does not need to mean turning away from caring, . . . A more important question is whether an individual has had the opportunities to practice caregiving that can provide a frame of reference for less direct kinds of caring in the future. Girls are encouraged to imagine themselves into maternal and caretaking roles; boys have less opportunity for this kind of exploration unless they have younger siblings. Once upon a time, too, the work that men did contributed directly to caretaking: hunting trips that took men away from their families had a very direct connection with the sharing of food, and the battles that men fought carried a direct sense of protection.

Today, the associations between jobs done by men and women and their care for their families are more obscure.

There has been a great deal of discussion of the need for fathers to be more directly involved in childcare, but the actual division of labor will always vary from family to family according to the needs and abilities of the family members. Still, caretaking, in its many forms, can be part of the composition of every life, and it is important to give everyone the chance to learn to care for another. Some children learn to attend to the needs of others by having pets; parents learn from each other and from their sons and daughters, if they let themselves, garnering knowledge they will use long after the childbearing years; the childless can seek out children to spend time with, building an awareness that can flow over into their other relationships. . . .

As we look ahead to longer and increasingly discontinuous lives, through which we can expect to move, from place to place and from task to task, it is clear that the congruence of different tasks, the recognition that a particular skill can be applied in the new context, is what makes the transfer of learning possible. Attention and empathy are skills, rather than biological givens for all women. Caring can be learned by all human beings, can be worked into the design of every life, meeting an individual need as well as a pervasive need in society. We need attention and empathy in every context where we encounter other living beings, and we need them to foster and protect all that we care for, laboratories and factories as well as homes and neighborhoods, fields and woodlands as well as nations and the peaceful relations between them. (pp. 156–161)

The centrality of caring to matters of health care priorities and policies and ethics has been forcefully argued, for example, in the following passage.

THE PRIORITY OF CARE OVER CURE

DANIEL CALLAHAN, Director of the Hastings Center, which he co-founded in 1969 to study issues in medical ethics, is one of the most respected experts on medical ethics. His works include

What Kind of Life: Limits of Medical Progress *(1990), from which this passage is taken.*

The pain and suffering of individuals should . . . always receive a high priority in the healthcare system. They are both essentially private experiences, even though we can often observe their effects. Pain may be defined as a distressing, hurtful sensation in the body. Suffering, by contrast, is a broader, more complex idea. It may be defined, in the case of illness, as a sense of anguish, vulnerability, loss of control, and threat to the integrity of the self. . . . There can be pain without suffering, and suffering without pain. In either case, only I can experience it, and only I can be relieved of it. Of course some degree of pain and suffering can be tolerated, and I do not mean to imply that the relief of *all* pain and suffering would be an appropriate goal for the system. It would not. I am only saying that they are forms of individual need—private, hidden, not directly shareable with others— that most merit our attention and that are most open to our help. It is the vulnerability that illness creates that most requires the response of others. I call that response one of "caring."

The term "caring" has its liabilities. It conveys, for some, sentimentality and softness, a vague ambiance of feeling rather than a systematic effort to make an effective difference. It need not and should not have those connotations. That in itself is symptomatic of the bias toward acute-care, high-technology medicine, with its comfortable presumption that it *does* something for people in contrast to merely holding their hands. Caring might also suggest acting by default; it is then taken to be what we give people if we cannot cure their disease or change their condition, a kind of consolation prize.

That is a biased understanding. Caring can best be understood as a positive emotional and supportive response to the condition and situation of another person, a response whose purpose is to affirm our commitment to their well-being, our willingness to identify with them in their pain and suffering, and our desire to do what we can to relieve their situation. . . . The caring response can take two related forms. One of them is constituted by the attitudes and personal traits we bring to bear, our concern, sensitivity, dedication, and steadfast patience, for example. The other is the way we socially structure our response: by organizing institutional support when needed, a support oriented toward the provision of comfort and security, assisting the patient to accommodate to his or her situation in some structured way. To care for someone is to give him or her our time, attention, sympathy, and whatever social help we can muster to make the situation bearable and, if not bearable, at least one that never leads to abandonment, the greatest of all medical evils. Caring should always take priority over curing for the most obvious of reasons: There is never any certainty that our illnesses can be cured or our death averted. Eventually they will, and must, triumph. Our victories over sickness and death are always temporary, but our need for support, for caring, in the face of them is always permanent.

Is there not something anachronistic, even archaic, about urging the priority of caring over curing? Does that not undo the very point of scientific medicine, that of finding cures for illness rather than settling for care? Not at all. The steady increase in chronic illness, the almost certain emergence of economic limits on many curative possibilities, and dissatisfaction with impersonal medicine press it once again to the foreground.

The primary assurance we all require is that we will be cared for in our sickness regardless of the likelihood of cure. Of course it is important for the healthcare system as a whole to know how it can prevent disease, and to know what it might do to cure it once individuals are afflicted. But above all it must be prepared to support and minister to people in their vulnerability to sickness and death, which can only be reduced, never vanquished. That is the one assurance we must all have from our fellow citizens and human beings. The greatest failure of contemporary healthcare is that it has tended to overlook this point, has become distracted from it by the glamour of cure and the war against illness and death. At the center of caring should be a commitment never to avert its eyes from, or wash its hands of, someone who is in pain or is suffering, who is disabled or incompetent, who is retarded or demented; that is the most fundamental demand made upon us. It is also the one commitment a healthcare system can almost always make to everyone, the one need that it can reasonably meet. Where the individual need for cure is infinite in its possibilities, the need for caring is much more finite—there is always something we can do for each other. . . . The possibilities of caring are, in that respect, far more self-contained than the possibilities of curing. That is also why their absence is inexcusable. (pp. 143–145)

———⟶⟶◆⟵———

Where the limitation of curative medicine in the name of the good of the society as a whole—which I believe necessary—courts the danger of an unfeeling utilitarianism, a simultaneous and counterbalancing focus upon individual caring can keep a concern for the individual at the center of the healthcare system. Caring is the foundation stone of respect for human dignity and worth upon which everything else should be built. Its presence can be a steady and faithful one even in the inevitable absence of resources to carry forward the open-ended enterprise of cure. It is in caring that we can address the uniqueness of persons, that which makes them different from each other. It is in caring that we can respect the claims and calls of individuality, that we can most show our solidarity with each other. When all else fails, as it eventually must in the lives of all of us, a society that gives a priority to caring in its response to individuals is worthy of praise. (p. 149)

> Writers have begged that dignity, empathy, compassion, balance, and hope be understood as essential components of caregiving.

HUMAN CARE

C. P. SNOW (1905–1980) was an English novelist and essayist. His writings include The Light and the Dark *(1947),* The Masters *(1951),* Homecomings *(1956),* Corridors of Power *(1964),* Last Things *(1970), and* The Two Cultures *(Rede Lecture at Cam-*

bridge, 1959). This essay appeared in the Journal of the American Medical Association *in 1973.*

Years ago, I had to pay regular visits to a friend in the hospital. She was a young woman of about 30 when she was first afflicted, or when the symptoms became manifest. She was clever, good-looking in a delicate fashion, and unusually kind. So far as it is possible for a human being, she was entirely benevolent. The disease that struck her was what was then called disseminated sclerosis, though nowadays the fashionable term seems to be multiple sclerosis.

It followed a classical course, with remissions in the early phases, during which she could carry on with her job. Total paralysis came more quickly than was expected. Sometime before the end, the most she could do in the way of movement was to touch a bedside bellpush. She couldn't light a cigarette for herself, or put it to her lips. Her speech was almost unaffected.

Many of you will know, better than I do, that this affliction, certainly in its first stages, is accompanied by a high degree of euphoria. Visiting her, I found that her room had been darkened and the hour lasted much longer. She was all set on cheering me up. It was hard to reply, until I got inured, and I never did so totally. I wasn't used to hospitals, and I hadn't seen anyone near my own age die a lingering death. I used to get outside the hospital in the cold London street with something like cowardly relief.

The euphoria left her as months and years passed, though she stayed in full consciousness almost to the end. I mentioned one hospital, but in fact she went to two, and for perfectly explicable reasons had to be moved between them. One of her pleasures, and acute pleasures, in the final phase was the knowledge that she would shortly be taken to the one that she came to love, as though it were a favorite hotel.

That preference had very little to do with the physicians at either hospital. For the most part, my friend was looked after by one physician throughout the entire illness. Her general practitioner, for we had solitary general practitioners in those days, had sent her when she first reported double vision and anesthesia, to a neurological specialist. I believe that he had some connection with her family, but my memory may be wrong. There was no difficulty, of course, about making the diagnosis and knowing her fate. He liked her, as most people did, and supported her, as far as any support was possible, for the next seven or eight years. That is, till death. He was a very good physician.

With medical attention much the same, the chief difference between the hospitals was probably in nursing. One hospital was quite accustomed to victims in this condition, the other, much smaller, was not. The nursing was good-natured, but amateur and rough-and-ready. My friend was incontinent in the later phases. One nurse said cheerfully, "No offense meant," as she dried up the bed, "just like my old dog."

This friend of mine wasn't one to stand on her dignity. She told the story with a sarcastic smile, as it were, to pass the time. Yet, even she had felt her dignity affronted—even she, and even at a period when she was passing into the extreme loneliness before death.

Many of you will know only too well what I'm trying to say in those last words. You have to watch it. Doctor Cooper, in a letter to me, has referred from the depth of his experience to the loneliness of each individual human being in serious illness, and most of all when near to death. It is one of the limits of the human condition. *On mourra seul,* said Pascal. I attempted to say the same thing in a lecture once: each of us dies alone. An academic critic thought that simple remark extremely funny. I wouldn't wish him or anyone else—and nor would any of you who have been compelled to witness it—to have to undergo the full extremity of that condition.

Personal Medicine

I want to try to extract one or two lessons and more questions from this experience of which I had to be a spectator. There are one or two factual points that are obvious, but where it is difficult to see the practical solution. Hospital administration, like any kind of service requiring trained and dedicated persons who receive little reward, is going to become an even more difficult task. It is already much more difficult than at the time I am speaking of, many years ago. Yet, while medicine becomes increasingly technical and mechanized, there is no substitute for good nursing. Surrounded by all the apparatus of a modern hospital—nearly all of which most patients don't begin to understand, being passively subjected to incomprehensible tests—the passive solitary human being is frightened. The climate of a hospital always has within it some wafts of fear. Those can't be gotten rid of, but perhaps we can prevent them chilling us too much. Like most things worth doing, it is going to mean money, training, discipline, and sacrifice. I don't know about your country, but in mine, nurses are underrecognized and underpaid. We could do with a new Miss Nightingale to awe politicians and administrators. . . . (pp. 617–619)

A UNIQUE CONCEPT OF NURSING CARE

YU-MEI CHAO is director, Bureau of Health Promotion and Protection, Department of Health, Taiwan. Dr. Chao is a member of the International Council of Nurses Professional Services Committee. This excerpt appeared in an International Nursing Review *article in 1992.*

Care is a universal phenomenon. Caring is essential to human existence, growth, development and survival.

Caring includes interaction between and among people. How one conceptualizes caring depends on what one thinks a "person" is, where this person is situated in terms of time and space and the relationship between the care-giver and care-receiver.

Therefore, how to locate a person who is in need of help at the right time and in the right situation is the major issue in the caring process.

The goal of nursing care is to support an individual's ego and integrity in order to attain this person's equilibrium. In Chinese, nursing care is called Hoo-Lee. Hoo means protection or surveillance; Lee, logic or management. From this semantic interpretation, a nurse's responsibility, in the Chinese sense, is to logically manage the patient's internal and external protective environment in a health-related situation. (p. 181)

THE CRISIS OF WOMEN'S WORK

SUZANNE GORDON is a journalist, author, and translator who writes extensively on issues of nursing, feminism, politics, health, psychology, and the arts. Her most recent book is Prisoners of Men's Dreams: Striking Out for a New Feminist Future.

. . . Those who manifest empathy are said to be engaged in a process in which they surrender their individuality to others and lose themselves in someone else's identity. In a society that values separation and "individuation," such activities arouse suspicion rather than admiration.

In the popular imagination, empathy is considered a simple, intuitive act, requiring only that you be a good listener. Empathy, many similarly believe, requires no more than reaching out a hand so that another human being can grasp it, or opening one's arms so that you can enfold someone in a comforting embrace. But empathy is far more difficult and complex. It is the attempt to put oneself in someone else's shoes, to stand in them, walk in them, and feel their pinch. It is hearing the different emotional or cultural language another speaks in his or her terms, without translating it into one's own. It is acting on another human being's behalf, doing not only what you want for another, but ascertaining what the other wants and needs. And it is learning how to *be* with another when you can no longer *do* anything to solve his or her problems.

This involves cognitive skills. It involves patience and it involves courage: in our *doing* culture, the *being* of caring is not prized, because to be with someone is deemed to be "doing" nothing.

To conceive, then, of caring work as an instinctual merging with the other is to ignore the discipline and knowledge required of those who engage in all empathic work. It is to ignore the fact that while women's work in the home and caregiving professions may have helped us develop empathic skills, empathy is difficult—sometimes impossible—even for many women. (p. 154)

THE JOURNAL OF AN ARTIST

ANNE TRUITT is an artist, writer, and University of Maryland art professor whose sculpture, paintings, and drawings have been widely exhibited and praised. At the age of 53 she began to keep a journal, now published as The Journal of an Artist *in two parts: "Daybook," from which this excerpt comes, and "Turn."*

While working on research projects as a psychologist at Massachusetts General Hospital, I had also worked there at night as a nurse's aide, and my feeling for the poignancy of human lives had been deepened more by this personal service than by the work in the psychiatric laboratory. In addition, released from the discipline of college, I had read widely and with passion and had begun to write poetry and short stories. These two lines of development had slowly, and without my noticing what was happening, become my principal preoccupations both intellectually and emotionally. The more I observed the range of human existence—and I was steeped in pain during those war years when we had combat fatigue patients in the psychiatric laboratory by day and I had anguished patients under my hands by night—the less convinced I became that I wished to restrict my own range to the perpetuation of what psychologists would call "normal." And in the light of what I was reading—D. H. Lawrence, Henry James, T. S. Eliot, Dylan Thomas, James Joyce, Virginia Woolf—I had begun to see that my natural sympathies lay with people who are unusual rather than usual.

I honestly do not believe that I would be an artist now had I not been first a nurse's aide. The evening hours are poignant for hospital patients. In the gathering night, I rubbed backs, fetched ice water, washed faces and hands, remade beds to smooth comfort, toted bedpans, fed blind patients, gave babies their bottles, combed hair, moved patients from floor to floor, and occasionally helped in the emergency room. I listened to low voices, harsh voices, screams and sobs, looked at pictures of families, reassured frightened patients and their relatives, prayed, washed dying bodies to make their transit decent.

Finally night would fall over the lined-up beds. We would dim the lights one by one, patting and smoothing as we passed. Care made a kind of family. When I walked through the dark streets to the subway to return home, I used to feel them all behind me, as if I were myself stretched out inside each one. (pp. 65–66)

THE SORCERER'S APPRENTICE

SALLIE TISDALE is a nurse author who, in her 1986 book, The Sorcerer's Apprentice, *describes the balanced involvement of nursing in a burn unit.*

Somewhere in this trial is a middle way, a balance of pain and compassion. Burn nurses find it or quit. It is a narrow trail flanked by extremity. One side, the side of empathy, is filled with wrenching sorrow, anger, and despair. It is where another person's pain becomes so visible, so inarguably present, that we attempt to take it on as we might carry a burden. This fails because, though we might succeed in weighing ourselves with the burden, we cannot actually take the weight from another: the burden doubles. We have *created* pain. And when we see another's pain (this is not as easy as it may at first seem), we quickly begin to expect the person to behave in certain ways, to respond as we would respond—or are responding—to the same affliction. We make demands of the sufferer, be it patient, child, a whole population. This is the way of the martyr; it is filled first with pity and then with contempt.

On the other side is a kind of total severance from the person in pain. This is more than detachment—it is actually a fissure within the person not in pain from his or her own memory and experience. Because medical science defines pain as physical, the clinician may not only fail to recognize nonphysical experience, but demand that it stop when he does recognize it. This is the World Series of artificial hearts, the unblinking preparation of the heartbeating cadaver. This is the undermedication of the patient in pain, for his own good.

Along the narrow road, where the nurses scrape little Michael's nerves [a reference to the debridement of a burned child], is a simple acceptance. Here is now, this is happening, keep walking. To project another's experience onto one's self (how would I feel; what if this were *my* child?) is both terribly necessary and terribly dangerous. Burn nurses work here year after year, anonymously, cutting off skin and treading lightly. It is easy to slip. They must help each other up when they fall. (pp. 129–130)

> Not all beautiful writing has been published. This final piece on *Care, Caring, and Caregiving* fits the definition of literature. It is magnificent in form and expression, as well as in its message. The essay exquisitely peels back the high-tech facade and exposes the raw nerves of an intensive care environment. It is lengthy, yet it must be read in its entirety.

CARING IN HELLISH PLACES

BETH PERRY BLACK is completing a doctorate in nursing at the University of North Carolina at Chapel Hill, with a minor in sociology. She has practiced in high-risk maternity and neonatal settings since 1981. Her dissertation research focuses on the emotional labor of nurses in the NICU, captured most compellingly in the following essay.

I love nursing. I love being a nurse. I have immersed myself in the profession of nursing for over a decade, caring for women in childbirth and for sick newborns, completing my master's degree, and pursuing my doctorate in nursing. My work in nursing has changed now. I am a nurse researcher. Nursing as a profession has a great proclivity to labeling its members as nurse-hyphens, I call them: nurse-managers, nurse-specialists, nurse-researchers, labels that define more precisely our particular work. But "nurse" retains its master status, linking the researcher, the specialist, the manager to her profession of origin. Preparing myself as a researcher in nursing has caused me to consider what nursing means to me, what I see as the essence of nursing; this essay reflects some of those moments of meaning, the essence of this privileged practice.

Nursing at its best is to experience with others the most important moments of human life—birth and death, hellos and good-byes, beginnings and endings. Yet with the triumphs of spirit and body over illness and death comes the certain pain of knowing: knowing that some patients will die and that some will not be allowed to die, knowing that for some I will cause pain in order to heal, and for others I will be unable to relieve their pain. I was required to confront my own pain in nursing, and the pain of those around me. The challenge was to create some distance from the pain, yet remain caring and human. And in acknowledging the common humanity between my patients and me, I came to understand that death is not always the enemy to be held at bay, but to embrace its necessity and its offer of relief. Nursing in a neonatal intensive care unit, I learned that those patients of the tiniest sizes face death in their early days of life.

I remember my first day in the neonatal intensive care unit. I was an experienced nurse, but nothing in that experience had prepared me for the first wash of raw emotion that I felt as I walked into that unit. I looked around, trying to make sense of the confusion of unfamiliar sights and sounds and smells.

There she was. A fullterm baby girl, weighing 8 pounds or so, was lying face up on an open bed. Much, much larger than the preemies that surrounded her, this child was deathly ill with a serious heart defect. Her color was white and blue. Her breathing was sustained by a ventilator that pumped rhythmically her life's oxygen. Nine pumps titrating minute amounts of sustaining drugs were suspended on IV poles around her bed. Chest tubes bubbled at the side of the bed, easing the pressure of air that had accumulated in her tiny thorax, the result of the therapeutics required to keep her alive until she was strong enough for surgery. A monitor at her bedside gave ongoing evidence of her status, continuously reading out her heart rhythms, her blood pressure, her temperature, all witnesses to the fact that human life existed amid the technology. Her name was Laura; only her head full of dark brown hair and long eyelashes gave her a semblance of being a real baby—a human child.

My knees went weak, and I felt myself break out in a slight sweat on my brow. "Oh, my God." I believed I had only thought those words, but Grace, my preceptor, said, "Everyone feels like that the first time they see a cardiac. You'll be taking care of one of those soon." At that point, I was not sure I would last another moment. "Soon" meant too soon. I would not be ready. What was I doing here?

I envied Grace's calmness and expertise. She had been a nurse for 7 years, and had gone to work in the NICU as a new graduate out of her diploma program. She was considered to be an exemplary nurse in terms of both technical competence and compassionate care. Being a preceptor on that unit required the nurse to be well-respected by her peers and the nurse managers: teaching the next generation of NICU nurses was entrusted to the best, the most expert of the previous generation.

Yet for all of her compassion and caring, Grace called the baby "a cardiac." Not Laura. Not "a baby with a cardiac defect." A cardiac. The baby *was* her defect, her humanity lost amid the pumps, the drugs, the monitors, the charting. A cardiac. I saw a *baby,* pale skin, long silky hair, long dark lashes on fat cheeks that should, if life was fair, be filled with her mother's milk. I was to learn that babies with heart defects are well-grown before birth. Their connection with their mother provides them with their life-sustaining oxygen and nutrition, and they grow big and fat in the womb. When they must become independent, in the early moments of life outside the safety of their umbilical connectedness, their hearts fail them. It was not long before I too called them "cardiacs."

The other beds were filled with premature infants of varying size, race, and sex. Many were chronically ill, ventilator dependent, unable to breath for themselves, or to take nourishment by mouth. Several were dying, one a tiny little boy weighing one and one-half pounds. Although he was several weeks old, he had never grown. A nurse was required to take care of him day and night, one to one, waiting for death that was inevitable, yet required to maintain his living with the latest in neonatal technology. His death was slow in coming; when it did come, it was met with relief.

I already knew the language of preemies before I began taking care of them in the NICU. I had had my nursing experience in a labor and delivery suite that delivered many premature infants each month. "Preemies are the enemy." It was our battle cry, for if a premature infant was born, it meant that we had failed in our efforts to prevent the birth of this child. These tiny infants, their bodies small enough to fit in my hand, became our failures incarnate. They were the enemy, ungrateful for our heroic measures to keep them unborn.

The nurses called them, or their mothers, by their weeks of gestation. Sometimes we called their mothers by their room numbers, at least in the private backstage of the L&D unit. Typical of our nursing report were sentences such as "Twenty-nine is a thirty-weeker on Terb subq q2, but I bet she'll deliver on you." What? In room 29, the woman was thirty weeks pregnant being given subcutaneous Terbutaline every two hours; the treatment was apparently not working, and the nurse believed the baby would be born during my shift. The enemy was coming. A preemie, a premoid. If it was really small, we'd call it a fetus, even though technically it was not a fetus; it was a baby, a neonate, an infant, once it was born. But to us who saw a tiny, gelatinous-skinned, match-stick ribbed baby whose chest painfully sucked in with each struggling breath, this was a fetus, born at the wrong time, of this world now, but not equipped to live here. "Baby" was reserved for larger infants, those who had a promise of hope to escape the trials of early survival relatively unscathed. The most premature were not babies, not in our language of the backstage. Oh, yes, we called them babies when we spoke of the child to the parents. It was their *baby,* what was to be the one they had dreamed of carrying home three months hence, fat and round and after happy phone calls to grandparents and friends announcing its timely arrival. This was their baby. It was our fetus, our preemie, our cardiac, our diaphragmatic hernia. We used words to reflect our need to be separate from their pain. And our own.

This language of nursing is important for it provides distance from the reality of the suffering around us, and it reflects the lack of control we really have over the course of these infants' lives. We follow doctor's orders, we don't write them. The language provides space, and hence relief, from the steady onslaught of emotional signals that come from one's self, one's colleagues, and the parents of these babies. The language of nursing in the NICU reflects the distancing that we do, the emotional work that prevents you, and protects you, from crying over each and every tragic birth, from feeling the pain of crying parents at the bedside of their sick child, from taking personally the failure to sustain these little enemies when death comes to them. Our late-night, dead-tired, tired-of-dead language was raw. Like Grace, I came to call the babies by their diagnosis. And worse.

Touch is central to nursing in the NICU. We touch to heal, but healing comes in many forms, and often we inflict pain in order to heal, to provide cure and to provide care. These touches include starting IVs in veins so small that sometimes you feel the crunch of the bone beneath the muscle as your needle goes in too deeply. These painful touches are meant to heal, to cure and to make better. On my unit, it was not unusual to hear murmured expressions of apology to the baby as we carried out these painful procedures; many times we explained to the baby that we did these things by necessity of physicians' orders and not by our own choice.

"They made me do this, baby. I'm so sorry." Maybe we were absolving ourselves of any blame for inflicting what was most certainly intense pain.

We tempered the painful, curing touches with gentle, caring ones. Babies on ventilators were not generally held, but when they were extubated, we would move a rocking chair close to their bed. There we would swaddle them in warm blankets and rock them as a mother would, singing to them, talking quietly to them, trying to make up for the pain they had endured in the early days of their lives, when they should have been held in the loving embrace of caring adults. Or maybe we were trying to make up to them for the pain we had inflicted upon them ourselves.

These caring touches were the sweet moments of my nursing in the NICU. Sometimes caring touches were done in other ways, gentle strokes on the small limbs of a bed-bound premature infant, eye patches carefully placed to block out the bright light of the overhead fixtures that were on day and night, sponge baths to remove the debris of illness, little touches to make a human connection between nurse and child. Caring touches humanized the preemie, the chronic, the trisomy 18. If our language was raw, our touches were gentle, aware of our capability to damage irreparably these tiny charges of ours. Sometimes we hated them, sometimes we felt nothing for them, sometimes we wished they would die. But we were gentle, because we were convinced that these infants experienced some goodness in their world through our touches.

Yet on occasion a baby was admitted to the NICU that some of the nurses found untouchable. I couldn't bear to touch Andy. I could barely stand to look at him, so great was my revulsion to this baby. Andy had a severe diaphragmatic hernia, one lung a mere bud that never developed because his gut, his stomach and intestines, protruded through a hole in his diaphragm into his thorax. Many babies die before this defect is even diagnosed, but Andy was "lucky." He had been "saved": an air ambulance trip took him to a distant medical center where he was placed on a machine that bypassed his tremendously damaged lungs, allowing them to begin to heal while the machine oxygenated his blood. He returned to our NICU to recover after his surgery, pale, clammy, his back arched from the brain damage that he most certainly had suffered. He couldn't tolerate formula; it caused him severe diarrhea that blistered his buttocks. His head was partially shaved of its thick black hair. His mouth was always open in an attempt to gasp for air, his cry was a kitten-like whine that never seemed to end. His eyes were dull. Andy suffered the ravages of his salvation.

Andy was my private hell. I recognized in myself an inability to get beyond my feelings of revulsion and disgust. And though I knew this sick baby was an innocent, a victim of attempts to make him whole and well, I absolved myself of any responsibility in that effort, and took care of him as little as possible. I didn't like what I felt for Andy. I didn't like myself much either, my inability to care for this child.

Other nurses liked the "technical challenge" of Andy. For some of them, Shawndra was their private hell. She was a very premature baby that, like Andy, suffered the ravages of healing. Like I felt about Andy, some of them felt about Shawndra. They couldn't bear to touch her. We never came to understand why we loved some infants and hated others, but we accepted that this happened, and supported each other through our own hells.

I could touch Shawndra. She was *my* baby, and I loved her. I took care of her for many weeks, watching this miniature human overcome extreme prematurity, staph infections of her skin and hip joints, fungus infections in her bloodstream, and drug reactions.

Shawndra weighed less than two pounds at birth; her parents were told that we'd do all we could, but her chances of survival were not good. Her little body showed the ravages of her short life's journey; after three months, Shawndra was in a full body cast required to support her infected hips. This same infection left one of her ears blackened and dead; it was removed. Her hair was gone in places where her head was shaved in a last-ditch effort to find a vein when she needed, yet again, a new IV. She smelled bad, her urine and feces stained her cast. Her skin was dry and peeling. I loved this baby, this little fighter whose will to live was indomitable.

I touched Shawndra when others couldn't. I would wrap her up in a small white blanket, turn the lights down and rock her for as long as my work load would permit. Whenever I had the chance, I sang to her and stroked the bare skin of her arms and face, the rest of her little body separated from touch, encased in plaster.

I wanted Shawndra to know gentle touch, to feel human contact that was soothing, and to learn that her world was not all pain and anguish. I wanted Shawndra to feel loved. I wanted to mother her, to do those things that her mother would gladly have done if she could have been with Shawndra daily: to hold and rock and love this baby when she looked unlovable.

Shawndra smiled at me one night. It was late, and a quiet shift, the lights dimmed, only the ventilators from the other babies breaking the silence. I held Shawndra on my lap, talking to her face to face. I always was surprised at the intense eye contact she made. As I talked that silly adult talk that grown-ups do to babies, Shawndra's eyes crinkled at the corners and she smiled a big toothless smile! I could hardly believe my eyes. Her face was beautiful and whole and healthy, filled with a baby smile that meant she could hear me, see me, and respond to the world with joy. Smiles from babies were like falling stars: they happened only rarely, you had to be in just the right place to see one, and they lasted only a brief moment. I rejoiced at her signal that she was healing, and from that time on, during those late night quiet hours that she had not yet learned were times for sleeping, she treated me with an occasional smile. I loved Shawndra, and felt proud of the way I had made a true human connection with this little child that others found so ugly and unlovable.

While much of the work that the nurses did was physical, much of what we thought was metaphysical. We talked of death, of prolonged dying in the guise of sustained living, and of matters of God. Our own religious backgrounds, beliefs or nonbeliefs, did not seem to matter much in the NICU. We talked of hell and purgatory, of being there and seeing true suffering, unbound by time with no end in sight. "Welcome to baby hell," we would sometimes tell newly-admitted infants, wondering what this poor soul had done in a past life to deserve this fate. Late night hours often made for strange theology. Yet out of this place, where the name was synonymous with suffering, true miracles happened.

Justin was one of those miracles. He was a full-term baby whose life seemed to end one night—pronounced dead by the flat wave forms on his pressure monitors—and we kept his little body on the ventilator, waiting for his heart to stop completely. Amid chest tubes, transfusions, increased ventilatory support, and every drug known to pharmacy and neonatology, Justin tried to slip away, his blood pressure gone, his heart rate slow.

His seventeen-year-old mother came in for the first time. Only one day after a Cesarean section to deliver her son, she was pale and weak. At first glimpse of her dying child, her knees buckled beneath her. Her mother and her grim-faced boy of a husband grabbed her by her arms and eased her into a nearby chair. This pallid and grieving woman-child wailed with pain, both of her body and of her heart. She saw her baby covered with blood and dressings and lines, the floor covered with wrappings and syringes and tubing and trochars, all evidence of our efforts to save him. But he hadn't responded, and his family came to say hello to the baby they had long anticipated, and goodbye to the child whose life was soon to end.

Then the death wait began. Overnight, over long hours, parents and grandparents came in and out, watching and waiting, praying and talking, asking questions. When will he die? We didn't know. What's taking so long? We didn't know that either. The nurses, and the doctors, thought he would be long gone by now. All of us waited some more. Morning came, and the night nurses went home, stopping in the waiting room to say good-bye to Justin's family. They would surely be gone by the time we came back that night, but they weren't. Twelve hours later, when I got off the elevator to go back to work, they were still there, and so was Justin. Refusing to die, this little boy got better without us. Once we stopped intervening, he healed. He healed. The nerve of that child! To save himself without us! It was exhilarating, and sobering, that for all of our interventions, this child got better when we gave up on him.

Two weeks later, Justin went home. At the NICU reunion months later, his young mom brought Justin, a well-developed, healthy nine-month-old, for us to see, and admire and to marvel at. Indeed, we may have been more aware of the miracle of Justin's life than she was. Justin had been as dead as a human can get and still live. He was a miracle even to those of us who don't really believe in miracles. He had escaped baby hell unscarred and unscathed. Yet miracles of that magnitude are exceptionally rare. I have only seen this one in my years of nursing. But knowing that they can happen sustains me when much of my work seems futile.

Death is the nurses' constant companion. The physicians don't know death like the nurses do. Death is the enemy of the doctors, who write orders to forestall death's work. We carry out those orders, but we become sensitive to signals that our constant companion is near, and know, usually, when he is at work. In the NICU, the nurses could tell when death was likely to pluck the next baby from its bed and carry it out of this life. The doctors were not in the unit around the clock like we were; they came back in to pronounce that death had passed through. The nurses knew when it was coming.

Death was not always the enemy of the nurses, since we believed that death was preferable to the life that some of our little patients endured. Death was painful for us in that it never seemed to come at the right time: too early or too late, after much waiting. And sometimes death would even sneak up on the nurses who were ever mindful of its presence.

Death came to Kamil too early and unexpectedly. He was recovering from heart surgery, doing well: his mother had visited him one evening and was making plans for taking him home. He died while his nurse was on break that same night. His heart monitor sounded, and we were sure it was a false alarm. But he was truly dying, and die he did. Vigorous resuscitation efforts could not get him back. Death was unexpected and too soon. This child was supposed to live.

Death came to Russell too late, after much waiting and anguish. He was very premature, and Lisa, a new graduate from nursing school, fell in love with him. She took care of him every time she worked for eleven weeks. That was how long Russell lived. Russell barely grew. It was clear very soon after his birth that he would not live, but we continued his ventilator, and his tube feedings, and his daily weighings, and all the blood tests and transfusions that the little babe could tolerate. We would warn Lisa, "Don't give your heart to a twenty-five weeker." But she loved him like I loved Shawndra, and took the risk of causing herself great pain by becoming attached to a little one almost certain to die. But we also admired Lisa's passion for this child.

Russell's death was slow. I was his nurse the night he died. Lisa had taken care of him on the day shift. She told me at the shift change report that she thought he looked terrible. He did. It was an intangible sort of terrible: there was nothing specific, he just looked terrible. The attending physician wanted to restart Russell's feedings at midnight. I told him that I thought Russell would be dead by then and asked him how many rounds of medications to give Russell when he began to die. The doctor laughed and said, "Just one." He didn't write that order in the chart. He wrote, "Begin feedings per protocol at midnight." And then he went home, leaving the nurses to care for this child that only we seemed to know was dying.

Russell died at 11:45 that night. The nurses and the resident doctor gave him five rounds of code meds while we waited for the attending physician to come in from home, so that he could tell us we had done enough to save Russell. We prolonged for a few more minutes 11 weeks of dying. His mother came over from the Ronald McDonald house and held her baby boy for the first time as he died in her arms. She sang "Jesus loves the little children" over and over and over to him. "My brave little soldier" she called him. The doctors were gone; the nurses suffered with her. We felt relief that another emergency in the unit distracted us from her pain. Death was long in coming to Russell, eleven weeks of suffering for this tiny baby, for his mother, for his father, and for Lisa who loved him too.

Our language of death was varied. For a tiny babe who didn't seem to know when to give up, we would exhort the baby to "go to the angels," assuring the child it would be alright there. Women who never set foot in the door of a church or a synagogue used that language, for there just had to be a place of peace and rest for these children, no matter what we believed of God or an after-life for ourselves. The angels would protect the baby. We knew it.

Yet some babies refused to die, or death eluded them for long periods, even when we knew that it was inevitable. Big fat fullterm babies were the worst for hanging on. These babies became sick usually through some indescribably sad birth accident, suffering brain damage that kept them from maintaining their own basic functions, like breathing. So they lay there, requiring a ventilator to breath, and sometimes dialysis to substitute for their own damaged kidneys. Everyone knew they were going to die. The only question was when. Sometimes it took a brave physician to stop the support and let the baby encounter death, but usually it took time—a lot of it—for the baby to become damaged enough, infected enough, toxic enough, or tired enough to die on its own. These babies we would encourage to go to the angels, for a few days. Then we would tell the baby, "It's okay to let go and die." Then we would ask it, after days of hanging on, "Will you just die? Please?" The babies that had some hope of living needed us! The angels were ready to care for those hopeless infants when we could offer them nothing.

So this is my story of nursing and caring in the NICU, the women who nursed there and the babies they cared for. This is my story, and I do not claim to speak for others. I love and hate that place, and I cherish the memories of miracles and human strength, and kindnesses and love. I also hold dear the memories of the pain, for the joy and the pain are intertwined and interrelated, one in sharp relief to the other.

The struggles for the nurse in this setting are numerous; the source of many of these struggles is in the nurse's position of being "in-between." The nurse is in between the patient, her professional obligations and role, the hospital that employs her, the physicians who order procedures and leave the nurse to carry them out. The patients, the babies, are in between life and death, sometimes more dead than alive, with only our technology to sustain their most basic functions. The babies are between their birth and the living of life. They are between their parents, who want to take care of their own child, and the nurses, who must take care of the child. It was within the walls of the neonatal unit, amid greatest pain and miraculous joy, that the meaning of the privileged position of the nurse became clear. For it is truly a privilege to glimpse the miraculous, to touch the untouchable, and to care for both the living and dying entrusted to me. That, to me, is the essence of nursing: the building and sustaining of relationships of trust and care with other humans at their most vulnerable.

VII

ON NURSING: THEN AND NOW

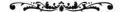

*N*ursing can be the means for transforming the human experiences around health; it can make a statement about human dignity; it can support human transition to higher wholes; it can provide a bridge to greater awareness and inner harmony. Nursing transcends politics, religion, cultures.

Em Olivia Bevis, *Toward a Caring Curriculum,* 1989

In *Notes on Nursing,* Florence Nightingale wrote about nursing, what it is and what it is not. This chapter could be described in similar fashion.

This is not a chapter on nursing history, as the title might suggest, although the importance of knowing our heritage has been emphasized, and the selections—some going back centuries—have been placed in chronological order. Also, this is not a chapter on an evolving definition or theory of nursing, although some of the writers might be viewed as having contributed to that body of thought.

145

In artistic terms, this chapter could not be compared to an epic mural or tapestry on which the influence of past events can be traced to the present. It does happen, however, that nursing's roots in the military and in charity are very apparent, because there is a richness of writing in those veins.

This chapter is more like a collage of personal experiences and meanings from various yesterdays and todays and from a diversity of settings. The fragments are of different sizes and textures and colors and intensities. And the pictures of nursing have been shot from a variety of angles, depicting early records of nursing, the experience of nursing or of being nursed, convictions about nursing, and emotions evoked about being a nurse. Such a collage might better be called "On Nursing: Then and Now, Here and There."

*　*　*

First, some selections from history and about history.

Deborah, The First Nurse Recorded in History

So Jacob came to Luz, which is in the land of Canaan, that is Beth-el, he and all the people that were with him.

And he built there an altar, and called the place El-beth-el: because there God appeared unto him when he fled from the face of his brother.

But Deborah, Rebekah's nurse died, and she was buried beneath Beth-el under an oak: and the name of it was called Allon-bachuth.*

35 Genesis 6–8
King James Version of the Holy Bible

---

*Allon-bachuth means in Hebrew "oak of weeping."

WHY NURSING HISTORY

M. PATRICIA DONAHUE

Many statements regarding the true meaning of history can be found in the literature, but the words of Sir Michael Foster, a British physiologist, seem particularly appropriate:

> *What we are is, in part only of our own making, the greater part has come down to us from the past. What we know and what we think is not a new fountain gushing fresh from the barren rocks of the unknown, at the stroke of our own intellect, it is a stream which flows by us and through us, fed by the far off rivulets of long ago. As what we think and say today will mingle with and shape the thoughts of men in the years to come, so, in the opinions and views which we are proud to hold today, we may, by looking back, trace the influence of those who have gone before.*

. . . . History allows for speculation and reflection. It can throw light on the origins of persistent issues and conflicts, thereby providing a basis for analysis that can potentially lead to resolution. History can open the door to storehouses of information that can be used to assist with the development of reasoned conclusions about specific phenomena. Critical thinking cannot help but be fostered and strengthened by the study of history. For one does not only seek facts about the past, but must think about those facts, discover relationships, draw inferences, and even call on the imagination to interpolate certain events. Facts themselves are bare skeletons and a compilation of them alone a fruitless exercise without discovering what the facts mean. How are they related? Are these new or did they appear centuries before? What guidance can they give nurses today? How may they predict the future?

Pride in nursing's heritage can be fostered through the understanding and knowledge of those nurses who helped to shape our nation's destiny, or at least the form of health care for our society as a whole. The fact is that many of the early leaders in nursing were involved in the social issues of the times including women's suffrage, child labor laws, public health, and national defense.

Finally, the search for facts, meaning, relevance, and truth can be an interesting and exciting endeavor. The study of nursing history can be and is FUN! (p. 77)

TRUTH

ROBERT PENN WARREN (1905–1989), America's first Poet Laureate, was also an accomplished novelist. This poem appears in Being Here: Poetry 1977–1980.

Truth is what you cannot tell.
Truth is for the grave.
Truth is only the flowing shadow cast
By the wind-tossed elm
When sun is bright and grass well groomed.

Truth is the downy feather
You blow from your lips to shine in sunlight.

Truth is the trick that History,
Over and over again, plays on us.
Its shape is unclear in shadow or brightness,
And its utterance the whisper we strive to catch
Or the scream of a locomotive desperately
Blowing for the tragic crossing. Truth
Is the curse laid upon us in the Garden.

Truth is the Serpent's joke,

And is the sun-stung dust-devil that swirls
On the lee side of God when He drowses.

Truth is the long soliloquy
Of the dead all their long night.
Truth is what would be told by the dead
If they could hold conversation
With the living and thus fulfill obligation to us.

Their accumulated wisdom must be immense. (p. 63)

GENERATIONS

LUCILLE CLIFTON is a California writer whose works include Good Times, Good News about the Earth, *and* Generations: A Memoir, *from which this excerpt is taken, and many children's books.*

Things don't fall apart. Things hold.
Lines connect in thin ways which last and last
and lives become generations made out of
pictures and words just kept . . . . (p. 78)

Powerful literature has been written by Florence Nightingale and about Florence Nightingale, the founder of modern nursing, who lived from 1820 to 1910. Miss Nightingale has written about nursing, the practice and the profession. The definition most often attributed to her appears in a passage below in boldface.

Nursing is an art; and if it is to be made an art, it requires as exclusive a devotion, as hard a preparation as any painter's or sculptor's work; for what is the having to do with dead canvas or cold marble, compared with having to do with the living body: the temple of God's spirit? It is one of the fine arts; I had almost said, the finest of the fine arts. (April, 1867, Letter to the Editor, *Macmillan's Magazine.*)

———

It is often thought that medicine is the curative process. It is no such thing. Medicine is the surgery of functions, as surgery proper is that of limbs and organs. Neither can do anything but remove obstructions; nature alone cures . . . . **And what nursing has to do . . . is to put the patient in the best position for nature to act on him.** (*Notes on Nursing*)

———

Let us be anxious to do well, not for selfish praise but to honor and advance the cause, the work we have taken up. Let us value our training, not as it makes us cleverer or superior to others but in as much as it enables us to be more useful and helpful to our fellow creatures, the sick, who most want our help. Let it be our ambition to be thorough good women (and men), good nurses and let us never be ashamed of the name nurse. (May 6, 1881)

I would rather than *establish a religious order open a career highly paid*. My principle has always been that we should give the best training we could to any women of any class, of any sect, paid or unpaid, who had the requisite qualifications moral, intellectual and physical for the vocation of Nurse. Unquestionably the educated will be more likely to rise to the post of Superintendent, but *not* because they are ladies but because they are educated. (To Dr. William Farr, 13 September 1866)

Our vocation is a difficult one . . . and though there are many consolations and very high ones, the disappointments are so numerous that we require all our faith and trust. But that is enough. I have never repented or looked back, not for one moment. And I begin the New Year with more true feeling of a Happy New Year than I ever had in my life. (January 1854)

Others have written about Miss Nightingale:

SANTA FILOMENA

HENRY WADSWORTH LONGFELLOW (1807–1882), a leading early American poet, whose work included The Song of Hiawatha *and* The Children's Hour. *This selection is taken from* Longfellow's Poems, *1886, and is the origin of the description (a lady with a lamp) by which Miss Nightingale became known.*

Whene'er a noble deed is wrought,
Whene'er is spoken a noble thought,
    Our hearts, in glad surprise,
    To higher levels rise.

The tidal wave of deeper souls
Into our inmost being rolls,
    And lifts us unawares
    Out of all meaner cares.

Honor to those whose words or deeds
Thus help us in our daily needs,
    And by their overflow
    Raise us from what is low!

Thus thought I, as by night I read
Of the great army of the dead,
    The trenches cold and damp,
    The starved and frozen camp, —

The wounded from the battle-plain,
In dreary hospitals of pain,
    The cheerless corridors,
    The cold and stony floors.

Lo! in that house of misery
A lady with a lamp I see
    Pass through the glimmering gloom,
    And flit from room to room.

And slow, as in a dream of bliss,
The speechless sufferer turns to kiss
    Her shadow, as it falls
    Upon the darkening walls.

As if a door in heaven should be
Opened and then closed suddenly,
    The vision came and went,
    The light shone and was spent.

On England's annals, through the long
Hereafter of her speech and song,

That light its rays shall cast
From portals of the past.

A lady with a Lamp shall stand
In the great history of the land,
A noble type of good,
Heroic womanhood.

Nor even shall be wanting here
The palm, the lily, and the spear,
The symbols that of yore
Saint Filomena bore. (p. 222)

NIGHTINGALE: THE ENDURING SYMBOL

MARGRETTA MADDEN STYLES, one of the editors and authors of this volume, wrote the following commentary for a commemorative edition of Florence Nightingale's Notes on Nursing *(1992).*

Florence Nightingale died 20 years before I was born, yet I have been enamored with her as long as I can remember. It's not because I have the need for a hero. It is that nursing has the need for enduring symbols. . . .

Florence Nightingale is our enduring symbol. Not all nurses will accept that gladly. For some she is the ancestor we love to loathe. She has been scorned on occasion by her own professional progeny as a crackpot, branded as a despot, even sneered at as a luetic. This is the venom with which we savage our could-be idols, so that we are left with no peers to look up to.

It is enough that we accept Nightingale for what she was and is. She was a person with strengths and frailties. She was powerful in her day. She planted the seeds of modern nursing. Her name survives and, above all others, is universally associated with nursing, by nurses and the public.

But more important than the fact that she *is* our most enduring symbol is the recognition that she *deserves* to be.

She represents many of the values we continue to hold dear.

The origins of many of today's nursing movements can be traced to the Nightingale legacy.

We are just coming to grips with some of the dimensions she ascribed to nursing more than 130 years ago. ". . . The very elements of nursing are all but unknown,"[1] she said then and may still be muttering to us from the grave.

I am not a historian, not a theoretician, not even much of a scholar. Perhaps I could call myself a nurse-patriot. But because of what I am and what I am not, I don't want to be a Nightingale student, to analyze her every word and deed. Let that be the work of others. I just want to believe in and draw strength from my impressions and to let my pride as a nurse take flight on the wings of fragments of her legend.

- I am staggered by the range of her intellect and interest. The same mind conceived and the same hands delivered the soft strokes of nursing and the hammer blows of social activism. Even today one can feel the bite of her determination.

- I think of her as the original liberated woman and take on new self-esteem in knowing that she rejected convention and comfort to clear the path for a calling then alien to the gentry. This is a striking personal statement about the importance of our work.

- I am proud that so early she brought rationality and theory and science—sometimes brilliant, sometimes rudimentary, sometimes mistaken—to clinical practice and health service management, proud that she has been called "the passionate statistician."

- I am amazed at her political cunning, moved by her militancy, and forever inspired by her stirring summons, "No system can endure that does not march."

- I smile that she was preaching vehemently about the environment, the community (or district), sanitation, hygiene, healthy living, and preserving the vitality of patients more than a century before primary health care was elevated to the rank of worldwide gospel at Alma Ata.

I am pleased that other professions, too, such as dietetics, various therapies, public health, and hospital management lay claim to her heritage. Yet I know she is truly ours. All of these are "elements of nursing."

These fragments pieced together form a collage of Nightingale as feminist, practitioner, politician, scientist, environmentalist, visionary, reformer—a striking, noble portrait. But I hold still another, a more personal, intimate picture in my mind.

Displayed within a showcase at the entrance to our school is a letter written by Nightingale in 1855 to the parents of a young soldier who died of typhus in the Crimea. She describes his last moments. I fancy that she wrote it late at night fighting to overcome despair and fatigue, after she had finished her rounds with the lamp that, in turn, became her symbol. And I fancy that she wrote similar letters to the loved ones of all of those for whom she cared so deeply and felt so profoundly responsible. And I am moved to tears of pride because I know that nurses everywhere are carrying on the Nightingale tradition in myriad ways and circumstances.

The Nightingale name is ours.

The ideal persists.

The lamp burns on.

The symbol endures. (pp. 72–75)

> Ironically, nursing, a humanitarian service, has stood out most nobly against the backdrop of a succession of wars and their destruction.

THE HISTORY OF THE PELOPONNESIAN WAR

THUCYDIDES. In 430 B.C., a year after the Peloponnesian War began between Athens and Sparta and their allies, a devastating plague broke out among the Athenians, killing a quarter of the population. Thucydides describes the pestilence in his history of the war.

Some died in neglect, others in the midst of every attention. No remedy was found that could be used as a specific; for what did good in one case, did harm in another. Strong and weak constitutions proved equally incapable of resistance, all alike being swept away, although dieted with the utmost precaution. By far the most terrible feature in the malady was the dejection which ensued when any one felt himself sickening, for the despair into which they instantly fell took away their power of resistance, and left them a much easier prey to the disorder; besides which, there was the awful spectacle of men dying like sheep, through having caught the infection in nursing each other. This caused the greatest mortality. On the one hand, if they were afraid to visit each other, they perished from neglect; indeed many houses were emptied of their inmates for want of a nurse: on the other, if they ventured to do so, death was the consequence. This was especially the case with such as made any pretensions to goodness: honor made them unsparing of themselves in their attendance in their friends' houses, where even the members of the family were at last worn out by the moans of the dying, and succumbed to the force of the disaster.

> Nightingale wrote voluminously about her experiences in the Crimean War. A few brief quotations, reflecting the power of her emotions and her expression, appear below.

I stand at the altar of murdered men. (Private note, 1856–57)

———>●<———

If I could only carry *one* point which would prevent *one* part of the recurrence of the colossal calamity; then I should be true to the brave dead. (Private note, August 1856)

———>●<———

No one can feel for the Army as I do. These people who talk to us have all fed their children on the fat of the land and dressed them in velvet and silk while we have been away. I have had to see my children dressed in a dirty blanket and an old pair of regimental trowsers, and to see them fed on raw salt meat, and nine thousand of my children are lying from causes, which might have been prevented, in their forgotten graves. But I can never forget. People must have seen that long dreadful winter to know what it was. (Private note, 9 February 1857)

HOSPITAL SKETCHES

LOUISA MAY ALCOTT (1832–1888), one of America's most famous women authors, is best known for her somewhat autobiographical novel, Little Women. *However, she was also a nurse and served the Union Army during the Civil War, recording her experiences in* Hospital Sketches, *published in 1863. Writing less than a decade after Nightingale described her experiences at Scutari, she wrote first about a day in the life of a nurse, and then about a night. Excerpts from the latter are presented here.*

A Night

Wherever the sickest or most helpless man chanced to be, there I held my watch, often visiting the other rooms, to see that the general watchman of the ward did his duty by the fires and the wounds, the latter needing constant wetting. . . .

I thought of John. He came in a day or two after the others; and, one evening, when I entered my "pathetic room," I found a lately emptied bed occupied by a large, fair man, with fine face, and the serenest eyes I ever met. One of the earlier comers had often spoken of a friend who had remained behind, that those apparently worse wounded than himself might reach a shelter first. It seemed a David and Jonathan sort of friendship. The man fretted for his mate, and was never tired of praising John—his courage, sobriety, self-denial, and unfailing kindliness of heart; always winding up with: "He's an out an' out fine feller, ma'am; you see if he aint."

I had some curiosity to behold this piece of excellence, and when he came, watched him for a night or two, before I made friends with him; for, to tell the truth, I was a little afraid of the stately looking man, whose bed had to be lengthened to accommodate this commanding stature; who seldom spoke, uttered no complaint, asked no sympathy, but tranquilly observed what went on about him; and, as he lay high upon his pillows, no picture of dying statesman or warrior was ever fuller of real dignity than this Virginia blacksmith. A most attractive face he had, framed in brown hair and beard, comely featured and full of vigor, as yet unsubdued by pain; thoughtful and often beautifully mild while watching the afflictions of others, as if entirely forgetful of his own. His mouth was grave and firm, with plenty of will and courage in its lines, but a smile could make it as sweet as any woman's; and his eyes were child's eyes, looking one fairly in the face, with a clear, straightforward glance, which promised well for such as placed their faith in him. He seemed to cling to life, as if it were rich in duties and delights, and he had learned the secret of content. The only time I saw his composure disturbed, was when my surgeon brought another to examine John, who scrutinized their faces with an anxious look, asking of the elder: "Do you think I shall pull through, sir?" "I hope so, my man." And, as the two passed on, John's eye still followed them, with an intentness which would have won a clearer answer from them, had they seen it. A momentary shadow flitted over his face; then came the usual serenity, as if, in that brief eclipse, he had acknowledged the existence of some hard possibility, and asking nothing yet hoping all things, left the issue in God's hands, with that submission which is true piety.

The next night, as I went my rounds with Dr. P., I happened to ask which man in the room probably suffered most; and, to my great surprise, he glanced at John:

"Every breath he draws is like a stab; for the ball pierced the left lung, broke a rib, and did no end of damage here and there; so the poor lad can find neither forgetfulness nor ease, because he must lie on his wounded back or suffocate. It will be a hard struggle, and a long one, for he possesses great vitality; but even his temperate life can't save him; I wish it could."

"You don't mean he must die, Doctor?"

"Bless you, there's not the slightest hope for him; and you'd better tell him so before long; women have a way of doing such things comfortably, so I leave it to you. He won't last more than a day or two, at furthest."

I could have sat down on the spot and cried heartily, if I had not learned the wisdom of bottling up one's tears for leisure moments. Such an end seemed very hard for such a man, when half a dozen worn out, worthless bodies round him, were gathering up the remnants of wasted lives, to linger on for years perhaps, burdens to others, daily reproaches to themselves. The army needed men like John, earnest, brave, and faithful; fighting for liberty and justice with both heart and hand, true soldiers of the Lord. I could not give him up so soon, or think with any patience of so excellent a nature robbed of its fulfillment, and blundered into eternity by the rashness or stupidity of these at whose hands so many lives may be required. It was an easy thing for Dr. P. to say: "Tell him he must die," but a cruelly hard thing to do, and by no means as "comfortable" as he politely suggested. I had not the heart to do it then, and privately indulged the hope that some change for the better might take place, in spite of gloomy prophesies; so, rendering my task unnecessary. A few minutes later, as I came in again, with fresh rollers, I saw John sitting erect, with no one to support him, while the surgeon dressed his back. I had never hitherto seen it done; for, having simpler wounds to attend to, and knowing the fidelity of the attendant, I had left John to him, thinking it might be more agreeable and safe; for both strength and experience were needed in his case. I had forgotten that the strong man might long for the gentler tendance of a woman's hands, the sympathetic magnetism of a woman's presence, as well as the feebler souls about him. The Doctor's words caused me to reproach myself with neglect, not of any real duty perhaps, but of those little cares and kindnesses that solace homesick spirits, and make the heavy hours pass easier. John looked lonely and forsaken just then, as he sat with bent head, hands folded on his knee, and no outward sign of suffering, till, looking nearer, I saw great tears roll down and drop upon the floor. It was a new sight there; for, though I had seen many suffer, some swore, some groaned, most endured silently, but none wept. Yet it did not seem weak, only very touching, and straightway my fear vanished, my heart opened wide and took him in, as, gathering the bent head in my arms, as freely as if he had been a little child, I said, "Let me help you bear it, John."

Never, on any human countenance, have I seen so swift and beautiful a look of gratitude, surprise and comfort, as that which answered me more eloquently than the whispered—

"Thank you, ma'am, this is right good! This is what I wanted!"

"Then why not ask for it before?"

"I didn't like to be a trouble; you seemed so busy, and I could manage to get on alone."

"You shall not want it any more, John."

Nor did he; for now I understood the wistful look that sometimes followed me, as I went out, after a brief pause beside his bed, or merely a passing nod, while busied with those who seemed to need me more than he, because more urgent in their demands; now I knew that to him, as to so many, I was the poor substitute for mother, wife, or sister, and in his eyes no stranger, but a friend who hitherto had seemed neglectful; for, in his modesty, he had never guessed the truth. This was changed now; and, through the tedious operation of probing, bathing, and dressing his wounds, he leaned against me, holding my hand fast, and, if pain wrung further tears from him, no one saw them fall but me. When he was laid down again, I hovered about him, in a remorseful state of mind that would not let me rest, till I had bathed his face, brushed his "bonny brown hair," set all things smooth about him, and laid a knot of heath and heliotrope on his clean pillow. While doing this, he watched me with the satisfied expression I so liked to see; and when I offered the little nosegay, held it carefully in his great hand, smoothed a ruffled leaf or two, surveyed and smelt it with an air of genuine delight, and lay contentedly regarding the glimmer of the sunshine on the green. Although the manliest man among my forty, he said, "Yes, ma'am," like a little boy; received suggestions for his comfort with the quick smile that brightened his whole face; and now and then, as I stood tidying the table by his bed, I felt him softly touch my gown, as it to assure himself that I was there. Anything more natural and frank I never saw, and found this brave John as bashful as brave, yet full of excellencies and fine aspirations, which, having no power to express themselves in words, seemed to have bloomed into his character and made him what he was.

After that night, an hour of each evening that remained to him was devoted to his ease or pleasure. He could not talk much, for breath was precious, and he spoke in whispers; but from occasional conversations, I gleaned scraps of private history which only added to the affection and respect I held to him. Once he asked me to write a letter, and as I settled pen and paper, I said, with an irrepressible glimmer of feminine curiosity, "Shall it be addressed to wife, or mother, John?"

"Neither, ma'am; I've got no wife, and will write to mother myself when I get better. Did you think I was married because of this?" he asked, touching a plain ring he wore, and often turned thoughtfully on his finger when he lay alone.

"Partly that, but more from a settled sort of look you have, a look which young men seldom get until they marry."

"I don't know that; but I'm not so very young ma'am, thirty in May, and have been what you might call settled this ten years; for mother's a widow, I'm the oldest child she has, and it wouldn't do for me to marry until Lizzy has a home of her own, and Laurie's learned his trade; for we're not rich, and I must be father to the children and husband to the dear old woman, if I can."

"No doubt but you are both, John; yet how came you to go to war, if you felt so? Wasn't enlisting as bad as marrying?"

"No, ma'am, not as I see it, for one is helping my neighbor, the other pleasing myself. I went because I couldn't help it. I didn't want the glory or the pay; I wanted the right thing done, and people kept saying the men who were in earnest ought to fight. I was in earnest, the Lord knows! but I held off as long as I could, not knowing which was my duty; mother saw the case, gave me her ring to keep me steady, and said 'Go': so I went."

A short story and a simple one, but the man and the mother were portrayed better than pages of fine writing would have done it.

"Do you ever regret that you came, when you lie here suffering so much?"

"Never, ma'am; I haven't helped a great deal, but I've shown I was willing to give my life, and perhaps I've got to; but I don't blame anybody, and if it was to do over again, I'd do it. I'm a little sorry I wasn't wounded in front; it looks cowardly to be hit in the back, but I obeyed orders, and it don't matter in the end, I know."

Poor John! It did not matter now, except that a shot in front might have spared the long agony in store for him. He seemed to read the thought that troubled me, as he spoke so hopefully when there was no hope, for he suddenly added:

"This is my first battle; do they think it's going to be my last?"

"I'm afraid they do, John."

It was the hardest question I had ever been called upon to answer; doubly hard with those clear eyes fixed on mine, forcing a truthful answer by their own truth. He seemed a little startled at first, pondered over the fateful fact a moment then shook his head, with a glance at the broad chest and muscular limbs stretched out before him:

"I'm not afraid, but it's difficult to believe all at once. I'm so strong it don't seem possible for such a little wound to kill me."

Merry Mercutio's dying words glanced through my memory as he spoke: "'Tis not so deep as a well, nor so wide as a church door, but 'tis enough." And John would have said the same could he have seen the ominous black holes between his shoulders, he never had; and, seeing the ghastly sights about him, could not believe his own wound more fatal than these, for all the suffering it caused him.

"Shall I write to your mother now?" I asked, thinking that these sudden tidings might change all plans and purposes; but they did not; for the man received the order of the Divine Commander to march with the same unquestioning obedience with which the soldier had received that of the human one, doubtless remembering that the first led him to life, and the last to death.

"No, ma'am; to Laurie just the same; he'll break it to her best, and I'll add a line to her myself when you get done."

So I wrote the letter which he dictated, finding it better than any I had sent; for, though here and there a little ungrammatical or inelegant, each sentence came to me briefly worded, but most expressive; full of excellent counsel to the boy, tenderly bequeathing "mother and Lizzie" to his care, and bidding him good bye in words the sadder for their simplicity. He added a few lines, with steady hand, and, as I sealed it, said, with a patient sort of sigh, "I hope the answer will come in time for me to see it"; then, turning away his face, laid the flowers against his lips, as if to hide some quiver of emotion at the thought of such a sudden sundering of all the dear home ties.

These things had happened two days before; now John was dying, and the letter had not come. I had been summoned to many death beds in my life, but to none that made my heart ache as it did then, since my mother called me to watch the departure of a spirit akin to this in its gentleness and patient strength. As I went in, John stretched out both hands:

"I knew you'd come! I guess I'm moving on, ma'am."

He was; and so rapidly that, even while he spoke, over his face I saw the grey veil falling that no human hand can lift. I sat down by him, wiped the drops from his forehead, stirred the air about him with the slow wave of a fan, and waited to help him die. He stood in sore need of help—and I could do so little; for, as the doctor had foretold, the strong body rebelled against death, and fought every inch of the way, forcing him to draw each breath with a spasm, and clench his hands with an imploring look, as if he asked, "How long must I endure this, and be still!" For hours he suffered dumbly, without a moment's respite, or a moment's murmuring; his limbs grew cold, his face damp, his lips white, and, again and again, he tore the covering off his breast, as if the lightest weight added to his agony; yet through it all, his eyes never lost their serenity, and the man's soul seemed to sit therein, undaunted by the ills that vexed his flesh.

One by one, the men woke, and round the room appeared a circle of pale faces and watchful eyes, full of awe and pity; for, though a stranger, John was beloved by all. Each man there had wondered at his patience, respected his piety, admired his fortitude, and now lamented his hard death; for the influence of an upright nature had made itself deeply felt, even in one little week. Presently, the Jonathan who so loved this comely David, came creeping from his bed for last look and word. The kind soul was full of trouble, as the choke in his voice, the grasp of his hand, betrayed; but there were no tears, and the farewell of the friends was the more touching for its brevity.

"Old boy, how are you?" faltered the one.

"Most through, thank heaven!" whispered the other.

"Can I say or do anything for you anywheres?"

"Take my things home, and tell them that I did my best."

"I will! I will!"

"Good bye, Ned."

"Good bye, John, good bye!"

They kissed each other, tenderly as women, and so parted, for poor Ned could not stay to see his comrade die. For a little while, there was no sound in the room but the drip of water, from a stump or two, and John's distressful gasps, as he slowly breathed his life away. I thought him nearly gone, and had just laid down the fan, believing its help to be no longer needed, when suddenly he rose up in his bed, and cried out with a bitter cry that broke the silence, sharply startling every one with its agonized appeal:

"For God's sake, give me air!"

It was the only cry pain or death had wrung from him, the only boon he had asked; and none of us could grant it, for all the airs that blew were useless now. Dan flung up the window. The first red streak of dawn was warming the grey east, a herald of the coming sun; John saw it, and with the love of light which lingers in us to the end, seemed to read in it a sign of hope of help, for over his whole face there broke that mysterious expression, brighter than any smile, which often comes to eyes that look their last. He laid himself gently down; and, stretching out his strong right arm, as if to grasp and bring the blessed air to his lips in a fuller flow, lapsed into a merciful unconsciousness, which assured us that for him suffering was forever past. He died then; for, though the heavy breaths still tore their way up for a little longer, they were but the waves of an ebbing tide that beat unfelt against the wreck, which an immortal voyager had deserted with a smile. He never spoke again, but to the end held my hand close, so close that when he was asleep at last, I could not draw it away. Dan helped me, warning me as he did so that it was unsafe for dead and living flesh to lie so long together; but though my hand was strangely cold and stiff, and four white marks remained across its back, even when warmth and color had returned elsewhere, I could not but be glad that, through its touch, the presence of human sympathy, perhaps, had lightened that hard hour.

When they had made him ready for grave, John lay in state for half an hour, a thing which seldom happened in that busy place; but a universal sentiment of reverence and affection seemed to fill the hearts of all who had known or heard of him; and when the rumor of this death went through the house, always astir, many came to see him, and I felt a tender sort of pride in my lost patient; for he looked a most heroic figure, lying there stately and still as the statue of some young knight asleep upon his tomb. The lovely expression which so often beautifies dead faces, soon replaced the marks of pain, and I longed for those who loved him best to see him when half an hour's acquaintance with Death had made them friends. As we stood looking at him, the ward master handed me a letter, saying it had been forgotten the night before. It was John's letter, come just an hour too late to gladden the eyes that had longed and looked for it so eagerly: yet he had it; for, after I had cut some brown locks for his mother, and taken off the ring to send her, telling how well the talisman had done its work, I kissed this good son for her sake, and laid the letter in his hand, still folded as when I drew my own away, feeling that its place was there, and making myself happy with the thought, that, even in his solitary place in the "Government Lot," he would not be without some token of the love which makes life beautiful and outlives death. Then I left him, glad to have known so genuine a man, and carrying with me an enduring memory of the brave Virginia blacksmith, as he lay serenely waiting for the dawn of that long day which knows no night. (pp. 47–64)

THE LEGEND OF EDITH CAVELL, BRITISH NURSE

JANE STILWELL-SMITH responded to the call for nurses during World War II, completed her training at Johns Hopkins Hospital school of nursing, and served in the Cadet Nurses' Corps. Further education led to degrees in psychology, speech and communications, and community and human resources. Like novelist Kurt Vonnegut, Jr., she believes "we don't learn compassion from technology, we learn it from literature."

In the dirt and stench and fear of the first
                    Great War
There was a strip of land between the firing lines:
                    No Man's Land.
The symbol for the Red Cross Nurse became
                    The Rose of No Man's Land,
Which gave the nurses great recognition for bravery
                    Under Fire
There was one nurse in occupied Belgium,
                    Edith Cavell
Who gave aid and comfort regardless of birth origin to
                    All the Wounded;
       Refusing to discriminate between friend and foe
                    Axis or Ally.

Refusing to obey the order from The High Command to
Cease and Desist!
Refusing the kerchief for her eyes when shot and
Silenced.
We shall never forget your legacy:
Caring without discrimination
Caring without disdain
Caring with love.

Post Script:
They forgot the poetic line
"The marksman has his moment;
The victim has eternity."

HELLO, DAVID

This anonymous poem appeared in the California Nursing Review *in 1988.*

David—my name is Dusty,
I'm your night nurse.
I will stay with you.
I will check your vitals every 15 minutes.
I will document inevitability.

I will hang more blood
And give you something for your pain.
I will stay with you and I will touch your face.
Yes, of course, I will write your mother and tell her you were
        brave.
I will write your mother and tell her how much you loved her.
I will write your mother and tell her to give your bratty kid
        sister a big kiss and hug.
What I will not tell her is that you were wasted.

I will stay with you and hold your hand.
I will stay with you and watch your life flow through my
        fingers into my soul.
I will stay with you until you stay with me.

Goodbye, David—my name is Dusty.
I am the last person you will see.
I am the last person you will touch.
I am the last person who will love you.

So long, David—my name is Dusty.
David, who will give me something for my pain?

THE SAUDI EXPERIENCE

MOLLY BILLINGSLEY is the editor-in-chief of NursingConnections *and associate director of nursing at the Washington Hospital Center, Washington, DC. This account of an experience in the Gulf War, 1992, provided by an Air National Guard medevac nurse concluded as follows:*

It is impossible to talk to veterans of this experience without sensing that they have undergone a profoundly life-altering experience. They all describe ambivalence about coming home and feel the need to stay in close contact with others who shared this adventure. In the larger perspective, it was not a unique experience. Nurses have been facing the terrors of war since Crimea. But, too often they have done it too silently, without the documentation they deserve. We as a profession also need this documentation in order to incorporate this very important group of people into our heritage. We owe them credit for putting their lives on the line, and we owe them thanks. The story needs to be told, for them and for us. (p. 19)

> The seeds of today's successes, as well as the roots of today's problems, can be found in nursing literature going back to the turn of the century.

A SUCCESSFUL EXPERIMENT

JESSIE C. SLEET (SCALES) was the first known graduate Black nurse to be appointed a district public health nurse. This brief account of her experiences was published by one of her supervisors in 1901.

I beg to render to you a report of the work done by me as district nurse among the colored people of New York City during the months of October and November. I have endeavored to search out the families in which there was sickness and destitution. But I have never hesitated to visit anyone when I have felt that a word of advice or a friendly warning was all they needed.

I have visited forty-one sick families and made one hundred and fifty-six calls in connection with these families, caring for nine cases of consumption, four cases of peritonitis, two cases of chicken pox, two cases of cancer, one case of diphtheria, two cases of heart disease, two cases of tumor, one case of gastric catarrh, two cases of pneumonia, four cases of rheumatism, two cases of scalp-wound.

I have given baths, applied poultices, dressed wounds, washed and dressed new-born babes, cared for mothers. When there has been an intelligent member of the family on whom I could depend, I have instructed them how to care for the sick one. When there was no one, as was often the case, I have made daily visits if the case required it, caring for them until they were able to care for themselves. Whenever I have felt it advisable, I have urged them to go into hospitals. Five of them received hospital treatment; two were placed in the Colored Home and Hospital, two in Bellevue, and one in the Presbyterian Hospital.

A number of societies, churches, and physicians were visited, the plan of work laid before them, and in every instance it met with their approval. They felt that it was a much-needed work and promised their hearty cooperation. Twenty-eight visits of this kind have been made.

Before closing I would like to speak briefly of two of the cases which have greatly interested me, and in which I have positive proof of good results: L—— K——, ——th Street, a young woman aged twenty-eight, complete paralysis of the left side; destitute, without any means of support, depending on her friends for food. After some persuasion she consented to go to the Colored Home and Hospital. Her recovery is very doubtful. The probabilities are she will never again be able to work and support herself and child, a girl of thirteen years. They have no relatives. The girl stands alone. No one appeared to have any interest in her excepting a woman in the next house, who has made it her business to be particularly nice to her, thus winning her affection and good-will. On investigation I found the woman is not a fit person to have a child, as she is not a person of good morals. I asked the mother to let me have the care of her child; this she consented to do. She was then placed in a respectable family, the woman promising to care for her until I could place her in an industrial school, which I hope to do early in January. I visit the home from time to time and am satisfied that the child is protected from those who would injure her. In this case I think I can safely say good has been accomplished.

B—— S——, a consumptive, twenty-seven years of age, with no means of support, a little girl of three years, and a mother sixty-five, lived in three small rooms, _____ Street. The three persons occupied the one room and slept in the same bed, the sick woman refusing to be separated from her child for a few hours. After I had visited the family a few times I succeeded in convincing the mother that she was endangering the life of her child. On my advice, she agreed to occupy the room alone, permitting the others to sleep in another apartment. A marked improvement was noticeable in other directions. The sputum was always carefully covered and a window lowered from the top whenever the weather permitted. The mother of the sick girl did not ask for relief, but that assistance be given her in obtaining work. I was successful in finding her work for ten days to do house-cleaning. The lady became interested in the family, and procured for the daughter the services of a specialist, who gave her every attention. The mother earned sufficient to pay a month's rent which was overdue, thus keeping her little home together, which was on the verge of going to pieces. The daughter, who passed away a few days ago, was made comfortable up to the day of her death.

Other cases might be spoken of, but the above is a specimen of the work which has been going on during the past two months. I cannot but feel that this house-to-house visiting, these face-to-face practical talks, which I am having with the people, must bring about good results. They have welcomed me to their homes, saying, "We don't know you, but we belong to the same race." They have listened to me with attention and respect, and if the advice which I gave was not always accepted, in no case was it rudely rejected. (pp. 729–731)

THE NURSE AND ETHICS

ANNE W. GOODRICH, nurse leader and educator. The article from which these paragraphs were taken was first published in Redbook *magazine, 1929 and later reprinted in her book* The Social and Ethical Significance of Nursing, *published in 1933. It was reprinted once again in 1973 on the occasion of the 50th Anniversary of the Yale School of Nursing, which she founded.*

To appease the great hunger for life of mental satisfaction, young women are, in increasing numbers, turning to the college. But the function of the college should be to stimulate, not appease this urge. One of the great scholars of the day, in discussing the purpose of the colleges and universities, calls attention to the influence of the universities, at the time of their inception, upon European life. "Here," he says, "the adventure of thought met the adventure of action."

To the nurse, working in the different levels of the social structure, in touch with the fundamentals of human experience, is given a unique opportunity to relate the adventure of thought to the adventure of action . . . . To effectively interpret the great role that has been assigned her, neither a liberal education nor a high degree of technical skill will suffice. She must also be master of two tongues, the tongue of science and that of the people. (p. 14)

THE NURSES' SETTLEMENT IN NEW YORK

LAVINIA L. DOCK (1858–1956), fearless feminist, outspoken suffragist, spent much of her career fighting for women's rights. A leader in all facets of nursing, she helped found what would become the National League for Nursing and the American Nurses' Association, and served for years at the Henry Street

Settlement in New York. She also wrote several textbooks in-cluding Health and Morality, *published in 1910, in which she discussed the taboo subject of venereal disease.*

Among the various "Settlements," so-called, in England and America, which are the outward expression of a unique modern discontent first embodied in the life and residence of Arnold Toynbee in the East of London, none is likely to be of more interest to nurses, especially to those who respond to other than purely professional notes, than the Nurses' Settlement in the great crowded tenement house region of New York. . . .

Its very beginning was out of the ordinary course of events, for, whereas today people who enter "Settlement" life do so consciously, the two nurses who, fresh from their training in the New York Hospital went into the densely populated East Side to live in a tenement among the masses of foreign-born people, had never heard of Arnold Toynbee; they did not know of Hull House in Chicago nor of the College Settlement in their own city, both already established, responsive to the same urgent pressure; they had not even read "All Sorts and Conditions of Men" in which Besant and Rice's heroine lives among the most wretched of London poor, and "Marcella" had not yet been written. In a word, they had no idea that they were beginning a Settlement. Simply, of the two undertaking this new strange life the one who was leader had, in the course of hospital work, learned with horror of the conditions in which the very poor lived, and filled with the conviction that if such things existed she must be among them to see where help might be brought, she persuaded a classmate to go with her and try what living among them might do. . . .

Let me try to outline the daily round in Henry Street. Breakfast is at half past seven, and unless guests are staying in the house, this is often the only meal at which the members of the family find themselves alone together. The postman comes: letters are opened and read, work and plans for the day are talked over and arranged. Afterwards the rooms are set in order; new cases that have come in are distributed by the head of the family, and the nurses go off on their rounds. The entire day is spent in caring for the sick; and in following out the different lines of work which develop from this, the primary one. The nursing is of course much like the work of district nurses in general, except for the entire absence of any kind of restrictive regulation. Each nurse manages her patients and arranges her time according to her best judgment, and all points of interest, knotty problems, and difficult situations are talked over and settled in family council. The calls usually come from the people themselves, though charitable agencies, clergymen, and physicians furnish a certain percentage. Often the nurse is sent for before a doctor is called, and then, if one is needed, she decides whether to apply at the Dispensary, or to submit the patient's case to one of the best uptown specialists, or to advise hospital care.

The patients being usually of a poverty which makes life a pitiful struggle even at the best, the nurses' care is freely given, with the exception of one who devotes her whole time to a service among those of more means, who would not ask for free nursing. This nurse's patients always pay for their nursing at the rate of twenty-five or thirty cents an hour. Beside the professional care of the invalid, all the circumstances of the family, so quickly learned in this intimate relation, become the nurse's interest, and, so far as is possible, her concern, and through the acquaintance thus established, she is sometimes able to open the door of a different life to one or another; to bring longed-for but hitherto unattainable opportunities within reach of different ones who had been by circumstances deprived of all for which nature had fitted them. As the Settlement family is quite a permanent one, its members entering for indefinite periods and never wishing to leave, the nurses form real friendships with their people, who call upon them in every emergency, year in and year out. In addition to her nursing, each one takes up some special work of her own according to her talent. What this may be will appear after luncheon to which we now return and where one usually finds some visitor or visitors interested and interesting, for no dull or stupid people ever appear at the Settlement. Those who come there have some work or purpose in life and feel a love for it in its various aspects.

In the afternoon, nursing work is finished, it may be in one or two hours, or not until dinner time, and the specialties are pursued.

One nurse, skilled in the Yiddish dialect, teaches a class of foreign-born mothers in simple home nursing and hygiene. These are the poorest and most hard worked of women and who have had the scantiest portion of the world's advantages. They have come from Russia too late in life to learn English, and can only understand their own curious jargon. They come weekly to their class, and after the lesson is over the samovar is placed upon the table and they drink tea. Visitors come in sometimes to sing and play to them, and reminiscences of Russian songs and folk-lore are revived in their minds. This lasts all through the winter, and in the summer the social part is continued in the garden. Another class is of English-speaking mothers, conducted on the same lines, and after they have had the nursing course, a series of cooking lessons in the big old-fashioned kitchen of the second house, where they sit down to a cozy, clean table with the prettiest of cheap dishes for object lessons, and enjoy the simple, well-cooked food made from the least expensive materials, and designed to show them how for the same amount of money that they themselves might spend, they can prepare dishes more attractive and toothsome than those they usually have.

These mothers are also of the very poor, though with more hope and aspiration than those who speak no English. They dearly love their classes, and call themselves the G.T.C., the Good Times Club. To those who know how sorely stinted in good times their lives are, there is unconscious pathos in this title. These mothers pay five cents a week for their cooking lessons.

Another nurse has for several years conducted a club of girls of fourteen and fifteen, the youngest in the ranks of woman wage-earners, and has given them in turn lessons in house-work, simple rules of hygiene and care of the sick, cooking, and physical culture, besides being older sister and adviser to them all. Another course of nursing lessons which is paid for at the rate of five cents a lesson is given in the evenings to more advanced young women and mothers of superior intelligence.

The nurse who is head of the house is endowed with all the social genius that could be required in such a life, and it would be difficult to enumerate the various branches of her activity. She is the fortunate possessor of a touchstone which reveals to her the best and finest possibilities of the natures about her, often quite unsuspected by those of less discernment, and this, combined with that best of all practical talents—the gift for bringing people and opportunities, the work and the workers, together—has enabled her to set free a multitude of energies, many of which strike their roots within the hospitable walls of the Settlement. The "lay member" who has had an unusually wide and varied social experience of the best kind, throws open her house to every demand made upon it, and is constantly busy in organizing some fun or frolic for the young people—a Kinder symphony, theatricals, recitations, or a musical party. A kindergarten occupies one floor in the mornings, the teachers of which are supplied by the New York Kindergarten Association, and their functions are among the prettiest that take place in the house. They have "mothers' parties" once a month, when the mothers learn the children's games and the ideas that underlie them. The "alumnae" of the kindergarten also meet once a week—tots who have been promoted to the public school but still love their kindergarten ways. Lectures find audiences there and many clubs, classes, and reunions come to the Settlement, being conducted by outside people, among which are classes in kitchen-garden work for little girls, cooking and sewing classes for older ones, debating clubs, a Shakespeare class for young women, special pupils with their teachers, and, for a year's experiment, a little shirtshop where unskilled sewing girls were taught to be skilled and capable of making a complete garment. A reading and study room for boys and young men is also in this house, greatly frequented, and particularly dear to the hearts of the Settlement is a club of boys led by the head workers, who study the lives of American heroes, and, under the influence which guides them, possess an ethical standard which would shame many a respectable citizen.

The "uptown" house meantime leads a similar life, and this winter a large school building belonging to the Children's Aid Society has been opened in the evening, with reading and game rooms for older boys and men, under the direction of the Settlement. Amidst the nursing and regular work that goes on, the social life is one of rare privilege and charm. Not only are interesting people from uptown and elsewhere to be met in the

Settlement, but all the currents of East Side life run through and across it. Most valued among the family friends are leaders in the world of labor—soldiers of the industrial army—both women and men, who come intimately to the house, and whose work and problems are household words. The poet of the sweatshops, whose pathetic verses have lately been translated and edited by a professor at Harvard, lived near by, and has read his poems there while men of literary fame listened, impressed and moved; young Russian and Yiddish writers come there, and aspiring young musicians full of talent and enthusiasm.

The neighborhood abounds with young men and women of fine intellectual gifts, who combine the hard work of the wage-earner with the capacity of holding their own in deep debate and discussion—in a word, here one has the opportunity of learning at first hand the movements and tendencies of modern life from the people who are working them out. Questions of municipal management, the schools and educational problems, industrial and economic conditions, the various directions in which social reforms are trying to develop; all these are being lived by the people who come to the Settlement, and this daily contact with the real things that are going on in the world gives an indescribable charm and fascination to the life. One seems, here, to be at the very heart of things. (pp. 27–35)

> Among more-or-less contemporary literature are many striking passages about the nature, importance, and experience of nursing in the late 20th century. The first two selections below are by a physician-writer and a journalist.

NURSES

LEWIS THOMAS, a physician and one of science's most gifted writers, devoted an entire chapter to nurses in his most famous work, The Youngest Science *(1983).*

When my mother became a registered nurse at Roosevelt Hospital, in 1903, there was no question in anyone's mind about what nurses did as professionals. They did what the doctors ordered.

The attending physician would arrive for his ward rounds in the early morning, and when he arrived at the ward office the head nurse would be waiting for him, ready to take his hat and coat, and his cane, and she would stand while he had his cup of tea before starting. Entering the ward, she would hold the door for him to go first, then his entourage of interns and medical students, then she followed. At each bedside, after he had conducted his examination and reviewed the patient's progress, he would tell the nurse what needed doing that day, and she would write it down on the part of the chart reserved for nursing notes. An hour or two later he would be gone from the ward, and the work of the rest of the day and the night to follow was the nurse's frenetic occupation. In addition to the stipulated orders, she had an endless list of routine things to do, all learned in her two years of nursing school: the beds had to be changed and made up with fresh sheets by an exact geometric design of folding and tucking impossible for anyone but a trained nurse; the patients had to be washed head to foot; bedpans had to be brought, used, emptied, and washed; temperatures had to be taken every four hours and meticulously recorded on the chart; enemas were to be given; urine and stool samples collected, labeled, and sent off to the laboratory; throughout the day and night, medications of all sorts, usually pills and various vegetable extracts and tinctures, had to be carried on trays from bed to bed. At most times of the year about half of the forty or so patients on the ward had typhoid fever, which meant that the nurse couldn't simply move from bed to bed in the performance of her duties; each typhoid case was screened from the other patients, and the nurse was required to put on a new gown and wash her hands in disinfectant before approaching the bedside. Patients with high fevers were sponged with cold alcohol at frequent intervals. The late-evening back rub was the rite of passage into sleep.

In addition to the routine, workaday schedule, the nurse was responsible for responding to all calls from the patients, and it was expected that she would do so on the run. Her rounds, scheduled as methodical progressions around the ward, were continually interrupted by these calls. It was up to her to evaluate each situation quickly: a sudden abdominal pain in a typhoid patient might signify intestinal perforation; the abrupt onset of weakness, thirst, and pallor meant intestinal hemorrhage; the coughing up of gross blood by a tuberculous patient was an emergency. Some of the calls came from neighboring patients on the way to recovery; patients on open wards always kept a close eye on each other: the man in the next bed might slip into coma or seem to be dying, or be indeed dead. For such emergencies the nurse had to get word immediately to the doctor on call, usually the intern assigned to the ward, who might be off in the outpatient department or working in the diagnostic laboratory (interns of that day did all the laboratory work themselves; technicians had not yet been invented) or in his room. Nurses were not allowed to give injections or to do such emergency procedures as spinal punctures or chest taps, but they were expected to know when such maneuvers were indicated and to be ready with appropriate trays of instruments when the intern arrived on the ward.

It was an exhausting business, but by my mother's accounts it was the most satisfying and rewarding kind of work. As a nurse she was a low person in the professional hierarchy, always running from place to place on orders from the doctors, subject as well to strict discipline from her own administrative superiors on the nursing staff, but none of this came through in her recollections. What she remembered was her usefulness.

Whenever my father talked to me about nurses and their work, he spoke with high regard for them as professionals. Although it was clear in his view that the task of the nurses was to do what the doctor told them to, it was also clear that he admired them for being able to do a lot of things he couldn't possibly do, had never been trained to do. On his own rounds later on, when he became an attending physician himself, he consulted the ward nurse for her opinion about problem cases and paid careful attention to her observations and chart notes. In his own days of intern training (perhaps partly under my mother's strong influence, I don't know) he developed a deep and lasting respect for the whole nursing profession.

I have spent all of my professional career in close association with, and close dependency on, nurses, and like many of my faculty colleagues, I've done a lot of worrying about the relationship between medicine and nursing. During most of this century the nursing profession has been having a hard time of it. It has been largely, although not entirely, an occupation for women, and sensitive issues of professional status, complicated by the special issue of the changing role of women in modern society, have led to a standoffish, often adversarial relationship between nurses and doctors. Already swamped by an increasing load of routine duties, nurses have been obliged to take on more and more purely administrative tasks: keeping the records in order; making sure the supplies are on hand for every sort of ward emergency; supervising the activities of the new paraprofessional group called LPNs (licensed practical nurses), who now perform much of the bedside work once done by RNs (registered nurses); overseeing ward maids, porters, and cleaners; seeing to it that patients scheduled for X rays are on their way to the X-ray department on time. Therefore, they have to spend more of their time at desks in the ward office and less time at the bedsides. Too late maybe, the nurses have begun to realize that they are gradually being excluded from the one duty which had previously been their most important reward but which had been so taken for granted that nobody mentioned it in listing the duties of a nurse: close personal contact with patients. Along with everything else nurses did in the long day's work, making up for all the tough and sometimes demeaning jobs assigned to them, they had the matchless opportunity to be useful friends to great numbers of human beings in trouble. They listened to their patients all day long and through the night, they gave comfort and reassurance to the patients and their families, they got to know them as friends, they were depended on. To contemplate the loss of this part of their work has been the deepest worry for nurses at large, and for the faculties responsible for the curricula of the nation's new and expanding nursing schools. The issue lies at the center of the running argument between medical school and nursing school administrators, but it is never clearly stated. Nursing education has been upgraded in recent years. Almost all the former hospital schools, which took in high-school graduates and provided an RN certificate after two or three years, have been replaced by schools attached to colleges and universities, with a four-year curriculum leading simultaneously to a bachelor's degree and an RN certificate.

The doctors worry that nurses are trying to move away from their historical responsibilities to medicine (meaning, really, to the doctors' orders). The nurses assert that they are their own profession, responsible for their own standards, coequal colleagues with physicians, and they do not wish to become mere ward administrators or technicians (although some of them, carrying the new and prestigious title of "nurse practitioner," are being trained within nursing schools to perform some of the most complex technological responsibilities in hospital emergency rooms and intensive care units). The doctors claim that what the nurses really want is to become substitute psychiatrists. The nurses reply that they have unavoidable responsibilities for the mental health and well-being of their patients, and that these are different from the doctors' tasks. Eventually the arguments will work themselves out, and some sort of agreement will be reached, but if it is to be settled intelligently, some way will have to be found to preserve and strengthen the traditional and highly personal nurse–patient relationship.

I have had a fair amount of firsthand experience with the issue, having been an apprehensive patient myself off and on over a three-year period on the wards of the hospital for which I work. I am one up on most of my physician friends because of this experience. I know some things they do not know about what nurses do.

One thing the nurses do is to hold the place together. It is an astonishment, which every patient feels from time to time, observing the affairs of a large, complex hospital from the vantage point of his bed, that the whole institution doesn't fly to pieces. A hospital operates by the constant interplay of powerful forces pulling away at each other in different directions, each force essential for getting necessary things done, but always at odds with each other. The intern staff is an almost irresistible force in itself, learning medicine by doing medicine, assuming all the responsibility within reach, pushing against an immovable attending and administrative staff, and frequently at odds with the nurses. The attending physicians are individual entrepreneurs trying to run small cottage industries at each bedside. The diagnostic laboratories are feudal fiefdoms, prospering from the insatiable demands for their services from the interns and residents. The medical students are all over the place, learning as best they can and complaining that they are not, as they believe they should be, at the epicenter of everyone's concern. Each individual worker in the place, from the chiefs of surgery to the dieticians to the ward maids, porters, and elevator operators, lives and works in the conviction that the whole apparatus would come to a standstill without his or her individual contribution, and in one sense or another each of them is right.

My discovery, as a patient first on the medical service and later in surgery, is that the institution is held together, *glued* together, enabled to function as an organism, by the nurses and by nobody else.

The nurses, the good ones anyway (and all the ones on my floor were good), make it their business to know everything that is going on. They spot errors before errors can be launched. They know everything written on the chart. Most important of all, they know their patients as unique human beings, and they soon get to know the close relatives and friends. Because of this knowledge, they are quick to sense apprehensions and act on them. The average sick person in a large hospital feels at risk of getting lost, with no identity left beyond a name and a string of numbers on a plastic wristband, in danger always of being whisked off on a litter to the wrong place to have the wrong procedure done, or worse still, *not* being whisked off at the right time. The attending physician or the house officer, on rounds and usually in a hurry, can murmur a few reassuring words on his way out the door, but it takes a confident, competent, and cheerful nurse, there all day long and in and out of the room on one chore or another through the night, to bolster one's confidence that the situation is indeed manageable and not about to get out of hand.

Knowing what I know, I am all for the nurses. If they are to continue their professional feud with the doctors, if they want their professional status enhanced and their pay increased, if they infuriate the doctors by their claims to be equal professionals, if they ask for the moon, I am on their side. (pp. 61–67)

WHAT NURSES KNOW

SUZANNE GORDON writes extensively but not exclusively on issues of nursing. The following was taken from a 1992 article in the journal, Mother Jones.

Attending to the human dimension of disease is far more than a feminine nicety. It is integral to the patient's survival. . . . (p. 42)

Nurses take care of patients twenty-four hours a day, seven days a week. If a patient with a broken leg complains of chest pain, it's the nurse who will contact the physician about a suspected pulmonary embolism. If. a patient with metastatic breast cancer comes in for outpatient chemotherapy and complains of dizziness, shivering, and simply not feeling like herself, the nurse caring for her will alert her oncologist to the possibility of cancer metastasis to the brain.

In addition to following physicians' treatment plans, nurses establish treatment plans of their own. They assess the basic needs of patients and do for them what they cannot do alone; they help educate people about how to cope with a disease or the aftermath of a surgical procedure; they become deeply involved—as patient advocates—in helping patients and families make informed decisions about invasive procedures or termination of artificial life-support systems.

All of these responsibilities mean that nurses should be major players in the evolving national-health-care debate. Yet to most of the public and policy makers, they remain virtually invisible. . . . (p. 42)

In a world transformed by women's liberation, nurses' innovations in care and their experiments in understanding the nature of cooperation and collaboration are some of the best-kept secrets of the gender revolution.

The need for a powerful nursing voice has never been greater. In a recent PBS special on the nation's health-care crisis, Walter Cronkite stated the problem quite succinctly. Our health-care system, he said, is neither healthy nor caring, nor even a system. A recognition of nursing's expertise and importance is critical to changing that.

Real health care, of course, involves far more than paying physicians to intervene when disease is well established or financing dazzling research into potential "cures." It involves education in disease prevention and health maintenance from childhood through old age, as well as providing skilled nursing care in hospitals when patients are acutely ill. A truly humane system would not push futile treatment on patients with terminal diseases, but would permit them to die in comfort and with dignity. A sensible health-care system that is genuinely economical would finance a cohesive network of long-term care to be delivered in the home and the community.

Nursing is already doing a great deal to inject some of these considerations into our disease-repair model. But imagine how these efforts could be advanced if we created a health-care system that valued care as much as cure. Working in collaboration with physicians, individual nurse practitioners would manage patient care, with quality—not simply cost containment—as the predominant criterion. They would identify those at risk for particular illnesses and recommend either immediate intervention or long-term monitoring. In health-care clinics, physicians' private practices, and health-maintenance organizations, nurses would routinely scan patient records to make sure that any recommended follow-up care was actually administered. Far from overutilizing health-care services, many patients—perhaps a woman with a lump in her breast, or a man with an enlarged prostate—may be afraid to return for treatment. Because quality care goes beyond regular office encounters, nurses would keep in touch with patients in order to schedule follow-up treatment and address any fears and anxieties, thus minimizing the chance that a minor complaint will escalate into a catastrophic illness.

Instead of depicting physicians as exclusively in charge of acute care, hospitals would emphasize the collaborative nature of treatment. Nurses, hospitals could explain, are the ones who have the time to clarify doctors' information and advice, explore the ramifications and side-effects of treatment regimens or high-tech chemical and surgical interventions, teach a patient how to cope with a reduced level of functioning, describe what will happen after discharge, discuss in-home care, and work with patients and families to help them cope with the termination of life-support systems.

Nurses, moreover, would officially be able to ask hard questions: Does an eighty-five-year-old man really need coronary bypass surgery? Is it fair to keep a patient on a ventilator, or would it be more humane to let the patient die with dignity? Could a patient be better cared for at home, and how can family and friends effectively provide that care? Most importantly, in both the medical schools and the hospitals that train physicians, the lessons of genuine nurse–doctor collaboration . . . would become a standard part of medical education.

All of these changes and many more, of course, would be reflected and reinforced in the political solutions to our health-care crisis. Nurses with advanced education would be allowed to prescribe medication and be directly reimbursed for the additional care they'd provide. Americans would be able to choose from a broad range of health-care providers—including nurse practitioners, nurse midwives, clinical nurse specialists, nurse anesthetists, and public-health nurses.

Creating the education, prevention, and health maintenance that would give nurses broader roles and greater financial rewards will indeed cost money. But these costs can be offset by limiting physicians' fees, curtailing unnecessary medical procedures, and eliminating the extraordinary waste of a private-insurance-based health-care system in which 23 percent of costs go for the administration of fifteen hundred different insurance plans. Ultimately, when expert nurses . . . are allowed to build trust with patients, teach people how to participate in the care of loved ones, or reassure a patient or relative who is deciding to forego treatment that merely prolongs death, they are saving lives and anguish, and money as well.

To create this new health-care system, nurses need to be far less humble and far more assertive in promoting their profession and its achievements. For this to succeed, however, they need advocates and allies—among patients, families, politicians, business people, and journalists—who understand that quality health care is dependent not only on heroic intervention and the promise of cure, but also on the efforts of hundreds of thousands of women and men who provide the care without which the cure would be impossible. (p. 46)

> One of the vignettes within Gordon's article is about learning nursing on a Native American reservation in South Dakota:

Nursing a Nation

It was a difficult week at Pine Ridge, South Dakota. First snow hedged in the broad, low plains with their pine-spattered ridges. Then came the rain that turned the snow and earth to mud. For the women sitting in a classroom in the barrack-like building, it was hazardous work crossing the dirt roads that join their small houses to the main road so they could ride the many miles to class.

These women are students at a very special school—the Oglala-Lakota College's nursing program. The school illustrates nursing's commitment to helping underserved populations, and these Sioux students are the ultimate example of a neglected population. The twenty thousand members of the once-great Oglala-Lakota Sioux nation are now scattered across a five-thousand-square-mile reservation that contains the second-poorest county in the United States. On the reservation, there is 75 percent unemployment and an infant-mortality rate almost three times the national average. As Michael Dorris's book *The Broken Cord,* and a television movie based on it, have so graphically shown, alcoholism is for many reservation women the only reprieve from poverty, and fetal alcohol syndrome the only legacy they leave their children.

To help these women learn how to care for their fellow Sioux and to make at least a small dent in the reservation's unemployment, nurses have tailored a school to the overwhelming health-care needs of the tribe as well as to specific scholastic dilemmas. The program, which began in 1986 and now has thirty-three pupils, is designed to teach students to practice modern nursing and medical techniques while utilizing the traditional Sioux beliefs about health care.

This effort to understand the context in which care is delivered is typical of nursing. The program's director, Judy Gaalswyk, explains that the school "teaches students to respect Native American health practices and to identify when clients are using them." This is essential to delivering effective health care to people who may often visit a doctor or nurse and then consult and follow the advice of a medicine man. It's also essential to understanding the difficulty patients may have understanding why, for example, they should come for a scheduled follow-up visit when they don't feel sick, or continue taking medication for tuberculosis six or nine months after their symptoms have disappeared.

The school adopts a flexible attitude toward its students' communal obligations in a traditional culture. The average nursing student at Pine Ridge is thirty-one years old and has 2.6 children. In order to attend classes, she may have needed help satisfying prerequisites in math, science, reading, and writing. For these women, schoolwork cannot be an exclusive focus.

"One of our students has six children," says Gaalswyk, describing a common situation. "She lives two miles off the main highway on a dirt road. Another mother has to travel forty miles to get to school. . . . For these women, sometimes it's a triumph just to make it to class." (p. 44)

The art, science, and excellence of nursing have been extolled by nurses as well.

THE ART AND CRAFT OF NURSING

DONNA DIERS is a psychiatric nurse, former Dean of the Yale School of Nursing, and editor of Image: The Journal of Nursing Scholarship. *A popular speaker and author, she has written many articles about nursing including the following from the* American Journal of Nursing *(1991).*

We do not allow ourselves to think that much about the art of nursing, and when we do, we tend to think of artful application, much like clinical judgment, rather than esthetics. But the search for beauty motivates the clinician as much as it does the painter or musician. Surely cure is more attractive than disease, and belief more beautiful than confusion; logic is lovelier than irrationality, and order is more decorative than chaos.

The art of nursing is, in part, self-discipline. Discipline is what gets us up at strange hours of the morning or night, makes us put on quaint attire and come eagerly to a workplace filled with demand and decision. Discipline makes a nurse check a drug three times even when it's the three-thousandth drug she or he has given. Discipline makes a nurse practitioner repeat laboratory tests because she knows the lab can make mistakes and the patient might suffer if information is inaccurate. Discipline is remembering that an IV down the hall is getting low, and discipline makes a nurse return to a patient one more time to offer succor when her own strength is lagging and the patient is shy or hostile or simply scared.

Discipline makes a person practice, as dancers or opera singers do. The tool of the nurse, however, is not the body or the voice, but the intellect, exercised on human problems and possibilities. If I only knew more, says the disciplined nurse, about electrolyte balance, or neurological function, or sinus-node activity, or the dopamine theory, or circadian rhythms, or cognitive dissonance. . . . If I only knew more, I could be better.

Nor is nursing practice a matter of learning the script of a play, then rehearsing and repeating it. A nurse seldom has the same words to say; nursing practice changes with each patient, each situation, even each heartbeat. The discipline of nursing is the constant attention to difference and unpredictability.

To continue the metaphor, nursing is choreography: In part, this means balancing demands gracefully, attending to the tunes others play, and moving in synchrony with the *corps de ballet.*

But on another level, the nurse as choreographer moves others. She decides what pattern and form are important for patients and then moves people, machines, paperwork, and decisions in what is very close to an aesthetic creation. A clinical nurse specialist moves a physician consultant slightly to the left, walks with the head nurse to stage right, moves the clinical investigations committee downstage, dictates the dance they will all do to the music chosen, and then stays out of sight behind the curtain.

The nurse-choreographer's talent is to create, out of the moving bodies, the electricity of conflict, the stirring music of commitment, a piece of action that is whole and intact, smooth and integrated, subtle as a minuet or rowdy as a polka.

Nursing is so enormous in its two missions—caring for the sick and tending to the environment—that no one metaphor from any one art can encompass it. But the notion that there *is* art in the practice suggests that there is also craft, in which the aesthetic is connected with the functional. The work of the mind in craft is holding a mental image of the finished product, then selecting materials, tools, and techniques to create it. Now it happens that we have words to describe the precepting model in craft: *master* and *apprentice.*

I always thought that one of our early pioneers, Annie Goodrich, encouraged nursing to turn away from an "Apprenticeship" model to an "educational" one. But I discovered that what Ms. Goodrich urged nursing to turn away from was "training"—the mindless, slave-labor approach once used in hospitals. She never advocated giving up an apprenticeship system.

I was delighted to discover this, because I think the master/apprentice model has a good deal of usefulness for those situations in nursing when what is to be learned is craft.

I think we should not throw out all there is to apprenticeship, only its slave-labor connotation. The craft connotation gives us another way to think about the nature of nursing's work and therefore the work of learning to become an excellent nurse.

Granted, the line between art and craft can get quite thin. In a recent radio interview, an artist said he sculpts, not carves, his wooden birds. He defined the difference by saying that he makes the bird that is buried in the block of wood come out. He isn't building birds, he's *finding* them by working with the wood.

To work as an apprentice alongside the master is to learn not only the craft but also the experience of *doing* the craft. Learning by doing shores up the novice nurse, who can believe that the work is not only possible but fulfilling, as the master shows it to be. The novice comes to realize, too, that the work is not random; it has shape and form, and beauty can be found within it.

These art and craft analogies point up what it is like to be a preceptor: The master is not teaching the apprentice to simply repeat the work of the teacher. Indeed, when this kind of precepting works best, the apprentice moves beyond the master craftsman to create entirely original work. The master's job is to help the apprentice shape her or his own talent rather than just to teach skill.

Skill is a much abused notion, too. Skills are thought to be the rudiments of more complicated things, and therefore rote, unchanging, mechanical.

But the acquisition of skill is neither easy nor automatic. Once learned, however, a skill is absorbed into the banks of memory and the fibers of the nervous system so it can be called up and counted upon with instant reliability. Carefully learned skills free the mind for analysis, for decision-making, for innovation and choice.

Skill implies mastery, but skill mastery does not define excellence in practice. It is only one of the springboards from which a leap to excellence becomes possible. (pp. 65–66)

THERE ARE RED LETTER DAYS IN OUR LIVES

JOELLEN KOERNER, Vice President of Patient Services at Sioux Valley Hospital in Sioux Falls, SD, wrote the following in a letter to the editors of this book.

Nursing is relational. A healing encounter within the profession of nursing transforms both the patient and the nurse. This relationship can occur over a period of time or with only one brief, but intense, encounter. Any nurse who has stood in that sacred place understands fully the powerful exchange that occurs when two souls exchange so deeply. I believe the essence of that relationship has been identified by Helen Keller.

> *There are red letter days in our lives when we meet people who thrill us like a fine poem, people whose hand shake is brimful of unspoken sympathy, and whose sweet, rich nature imparts on our eager, impatient spirit a wonderful restfulness which, in its essence, is divine. Perhaps we never saw them before, and they may never cross our life path again, but the influence of their calm, mellow nature is a libation poured upon our discontent, and we feel its healing touch, as the ocean feels the mountain stream freshening its brim.*

This, I believe, is the essence of nursing.

> Through literature, nurses have sought to rally one another around the variegated splendor—both earthy and lofty—of their profession.

HOW CAN YOU BEAR TO BE A NURSE?

MARY B. MALLISON wrote this editorial for the American Journal of Nursing *in 1987.*

National Nurses' Day is May 6 this year. No doubt people will ask you some of these questions. Please add to this list and send us your answers, will you?

How can you be a nurse? How can you bear the sight of blood?

Wait until you slide a catheter into a tiny vein just before it collapses. The flashback of blood you see will make you sing.

How can you be a nurse? How can you bear the sight, the embarrassment, of urine?

Wait until your new postpartum patient can't void, and her uterus is rising. Your persistent maneuvers finally work, making a catheter unnecessary. Urine then looks glorious.

How can you be a nurse? How can you bear to touch that alcoholic who hasn't had a bath in weeks?

Wait until you've repeatedly given ice lavages to that alcoholic and his esophageal varices have finally stopped bleeding. When he actually recovers enough to amble onto your unit to visit, dirt and all, you'll be happy enough to hug him.

How can you be a nurse? How can you bear to watch someone die?

Wait until you've worked for weeks helping a dying woman repair a decades-old conflict with her children, and at some point along the way you see the guilt fall from their shoulders and peace enter her eyes. Watching such a death can be an exaltation.

How can you be a nurse? How can you bear the sight and smell of feces?

Wait until you've been anxious about the diarrhea that nothing has stopped in an AIDS patient. Finally, your strategies work and you see and smell normal stool. You'll welcome that smell.

How can you be a nurse? How can you bear to watch children suffer?

Wait until you've rocked and soothed a suffering child into peaceful sleep, and you feel the child's relief washing over you like a blessing. Then you won't need to ask.

How can you be a nurse? How can you bear to look at searing trauma, at burned people?

Wait until you see healthy granulation tissue that has been given a chance because your sensitive nose detected an infection before it could take hold. That healing will look beautiful to you.

How can you be a nurse? How can you bear the stream of abusive words heaped on you by psychotic patients?

Wait until you've prodded and pulled a silent, withdrawn catatonic back over the lifeline, and she releases a string of expletives. Could Mozart sound better?

How can you be a nurse? How can you bear the sound of babies crying?

Wait until your combination of vigilance, bulldog advocacy, and gentle handling has given a preemie's lungs the time they needed to develop, and you hear his first lusty cry. You'll laugh out loud!

How can you be a nurse? How can you bear to care for frustrating, confused Alzheimer's patients?

Wait until you've devised a combination of strategies that provide exercise and permit safe wandering, and you see a lift, almost a spring, in a patient's shuffling gait. You'll feel the lightness of Baryshnikov in your own step that day.

How can you be a nurse? So many of your patients are so old, so sick, these days. How can you bear the thought that, in the end, your care may make no difference?

Wait until you've used your hands and eyes and voice to dispel terror, to show a helpless person that his life is respected, that he has dignity. Your caring helps him care about himself. His helplessness forces you to think about the brevity of your own life.

Then and there, you decide yet again to reject the pallid pastel life. No tepid sail across a protected cove for you. No easy answers.

So you keep choosing to be a nurse. You have days of frustration, nights of despair, terrible angers. Your highs and lows are peaks and chasms, not hills and valleys. The defeats come more than often enough to keep you humble: the problems you can't untangle, the lives that seep away too fast, the meanings that elude your understanding.

But you keep working at it, learning from it, knowing the next peak lies ahead.

And gradually you realize your palette is filling up with colors. You see more shades of meaning. You laugh more. You realize you are

well on your way to creating a work of art, maybe even a masterpiece. So that's why you remained a nurse. To your surprise, your
greatest work of art is turning out to be your own life. (p. 419)

A KALEIDOSCOPIC VIEW OF NURSING

*CYNTHIA M. FREUND is currently the Dean at the School of Nurs-
ing of the University of North Carolina—Chapel Hill. This excerpt is taken from her 1990 book,* The Unity of Education,
Research, and Practice.

Unity is a state of mind that I have described as "professional
solidarity." . . . I chose the word *solidarity,* as opposed to *unity,*
deliberately. When we think of solidarity movements (such as
the solidarity movement that began in Poland and spread to
other eastern European countries and South Africa), we think of
individuals who risk their livelihood and very existence to support a cause that will, in the long run, benefit the whole. Individual interests, which may be as basic as food on the table or life
itself, are subsumed in favor of a greater good.

I am not suggesting that we need to risk the well-being of our
families or our very lives to achieve our goals as a profession
and to be united in caring for nursing—professional solidarity
will not demand that from us. I am suggesting that solidarity, for
us, is a state of mind—it is like citizenship. We belong to a plural-
istic society and our citizenship implies our endorsement of pluralism. We vote on issues, we elect people to represent us and
make decisions for us (for the benefit of the *whole),* and we hope
that, more often than not, *we* are the whole—that *we* benefit. We
know, of course, that our country has done and will do things
with which we may not agree as an individual, and that our rep-
resentatives will make decisions for the benefit of the whole that
do not benefit us as individuals—but we do not renounce our citizenship; we do not drop out of the societal collective. We may
fight, campaign, and work to change that with which we do not
agree; we may also disagree with decisions, yet choose to do
nothing. If we felt morally indignant or outraged, we might revolt

or move to another country, but short of that, we hang in there—in the spirit of citizenship and in support of the principles of pluralism and solidarity.

If all of us who call ourselves nurses would view our profession with a similar spirit of solidarity, we would be united in caring for nursing. Professional solidarity is a commitment to our profession and its goals. It is support of the whole, rather than of individual interests. It is an exquisite professional state of mind. United in caring for nursing, in the global context of caring, means preserving this profession we all care about. United in caring for nursing means respecting and valuing every nurse's contribution, disenfranchising none, recognizing that we all depend on each other, and knowing that the collective contribution of nursing to society is greater than the sum of its parts. Debate, differing opinion, diversity (in practice settings and levels of practice, in education, and in research) are vital—they are the lifeblood of our profession.

Our diversity is our richness—it is our kaleidoscope, and each and every twist results in a unified and beautiful pattern that we know as nursing. Unity is invisible, like the intricate web of lines that guide the crystals in a kaleidoscopic pattern. Think of each and every crystal in a kaleidoscope as representing you, me, the person next to you . . . all nurses. Think of the entire pattern as all of nursing—the profession of nursing. Look at the pattern—it may appear to have sections; there may be boundaries between crystals—then twist the kaleidoscope. The crystals (you and I) move and change from one section to another, and we may see new boundaries.

In the kaleidoscopic pattern of nursing, we create many artificial boundaries for convenience to describe nursing, like the boundaries between practice, research, and education; the boundaries between practice in different settings; the boundaries between clinical, systems, and policy research; the boundaries between levels of educational programs; and the boundaries between technical, professional, and advanced practice, for example. Artificial boundaries of convenience soon take on meaning beyond their intention—they become great walls (and sometimes war zones), surrounded by ideologies, rhetoric, and dogma. When we think we are divided, we lose sight of the unique and valuable contributions each and every nurse, in each and every way, makes to the profession. Nursing practice is the heart and soul of nursing; it is through nursing practice that we fulfill our mandate to society. Education and research exist to serve the profession—education prepares nurses for practice, and research informs practice and documents nurses' contributions to the health of society. In this we are all united—in one kaleidoscopic pattern. (pp. 22–24)

AGENDA FOR CHANGE

PATRICIA MOCCIA, co-editor and co-author of this volume, is the Acting Director of the National League for Nurses. This excerpt is taken from her 1988 work, Curriculum Revolution: Agenda for Change.

We are faced with many choices as we decide whether to join the procession of educated men and how to choose between the high ground or the swamp. Should we adopt the values of commerce and redesign health care systems accordingly? Should we accept competition as the modus operandi or insist on other measures for people in need? How do we decide who will be cared for and who will not? Who will pay and how much?

. . . Perhaps it is time for us to turn away from the exchange between buyers and sellers, providers and consumers, and turn back to an exchange between two people trying to understand the space they share. Perhaps it is time for us to enter into dialogue with patients, since they are the ones most affected by these questions. Perhaps it is time for us to hear their call and respond authentically; perhaps it is time they were permitted to hear ours. And perhaps it is time to teach our students this.

. . . Only when we grant love, passion, feeling, and imagination the same legitimacy that we grant reason, logic, and techniques;

only when we restore our sense of community and reclaim our place as active participants in our world; only then will we be healthy as individuals, a profession, and a world community.

Now that we know what to do intellectually, we must commit our love and our passions to doing it. (p. 63)

Note

1. Nightingale, F. (1859). *Notes on nursing: What it is, and what it is not,* p. 6. London: Harrison & Sons.

VIII

ON LIFE STAGES

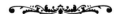

*F*irst, potential life is everywhere. Land that looks barren and wasted, branches that look dead, a bush that looks scraggly, all of a sudden explode into life.

Second, life takes many different forms . . . of size and shape and color and smell and texture . . . forms of movement and growth . . . Judgment about . . . . how different forms of life declare their being seems arrogant, presumptuous.

Third, **there are different stages of life. Each is part of a whole process . . . . Growth is the process, not the product.**

Fourth, when living things are uprooted, there is danger that they won't survive . . . it's hard to go from one environment, even a bad, cramped, stuffy chaotic environment to another, even if the other is open and roomy and sunny . . . . Exposed roots are very, very vulnerable.

Bernice Mennis, *Gardens, Growth, & Community,* 1977

How do health and illness and caretaking appear through the looking glass of life stages? Fragments of literature, like crystal, enable us to penetrate each stage and, when fitted together, reveal life as one piece, one creation. The selections in this chapter have been clustered and presented in this order: pregnancy, birth, parenthood; childhood; families; and aging.

*   *   *

PREGNANCY, BIRTH, PARENTHOOD

Pregnancy is such an utterly specific condition, yet also one that is a part of the most general rhythm of life that there is. . . . During pregnancy one senses a profound harmony with the universe, an interchange between the grand and the particular which endows every detail of life with new vividness and meaning.

Suzanna Lessard, *The New Yorker,* 1980

Birth usually feels like a steamy kitchen—similar to holiday preparations, except that the smells are different. The smell of sweat is more acrid, there are some fetid odors, there is the smell and steam rising from the blood. The air is thick, pungent, fertile. It is hard not to be reminded of fresh straw and night stars. There is near and heady promise.

Penny Armstrong, *A Midwife's Story,* 1986

THE ESSENCE OF MIDWIFERY

LINDA V. WALSH was assistant program director of the Nurse Midwifery Program at the University of Pennsylvania and a doctoral student in nursing at that institution when this was written. Her research focused on nurse midwifery practice in the early 20th century.

He who uttered the words "Routine Delivery"
Or hastily wrote "Normal Spontaneous Delivery" as

one further procedure in a busy day
Couldn't have really been with her.
He couldn't have been
Or he would have felt her muscles as they
    worked
    strained
    pushed
that infant into the world.
He couldn't have been,
Or he would have truly felt her perspiration weep from
    her body as she reached for strength deep
    within.
No, he couldn't have really been with her.
If he were, he would have appreciated her expression
    as it changed from excitement, to concentration,
    to fear, and to excitement and peace.
He couldn't have held her,
Whispering
    "You're almost there"
    "You're doing so beautifully"
    "You are so strong."
Routine delivery.
He couldn't have been there.
He couldn't have taken the time
to pause in awe and wonder
as that little head came slowly, ever so slowly,
and the eyes opened and looked out with such trust
    and wisdom.
Procedure—normal spontaneous delivery.
He couldn't have been with her.
He couldn't have marveled as she reached down,
    drawing her daughter to her breast
Laughing, shouting, crying—all the emotions of birth.
No, he couldn't have been with her.
For she who has been with woman knows there is no
    routine birth, and that delivery is not a
    procedure.
Being with woman is opening up,

sharing,
loving,
caring.
Being with woman is truly being a midwife.

THE GIFT

CAROL BAKER HANSEN lived in Newcastle, Maine, and was an editorial assistant at Bowdoin College when this poem was written. It was published in Balancing Act: A Book of Poems by Maine Women. *Her poems have also appeared in* The Nation, North American Review, *and other journals.*

"Here's your baby, Mrs. Hansen,"
says the girl from the nursery with what
looks like just a blanket
tucked in the crook of her right arm.

Mine? My baby? I go along
with the charade as she checks
my armband against
the baby's footband and hands me

the blanket. Mother of God.
There is a lotus a sunburst a perfect
face resting in the white curve
of cotton, glowing, lit from within.

Mine. A gift then? Surely
I did not earn this miracle
by that pumping my body did,
by that last show of good blood.

She is sleeping. Her lids are lavender.
Perhaps she is blind like kittens.
Surely this roseflesh fruitsoft
babyskin belongs to no one. I am

only the pitcher that poured her out,
pot she took root in, oven she rose in.

She, the pure germ a gnome found
locked at the heart of a wrinkled tuber.

She wakes and takes my breast,
now so round and full of light,
and sucks, and we
pretend I am her mother.

THE RAIN AND THEIR DREAMS

*BEATRICE CROFTS YORKER is a nurse attorney who is Chair of
Psychiatric/Mental Health Nursing at Georgia State University
in Atlanta. This poem was published in* The Journal of Child
and Adolescent Psychopharmacology *in 1991.*

She felt
From his birth
He was different.
One would never guess
From outward appearances
His eyes
Clear as a summer lake
Every feature perfectly sculpted
Gave her some comfort.
The chaos in his gaze.
The chasm
Her murmurs and tender words fell into
Before they reached his ears

She treasured the early morning times
While he still slept
She crept close
He would let her love him
A brief moment
Until he recoiled.

The "Helping Place" welcomed
And whisked him away.
They smiled

Hours of skilled thought
Nodding and knowing

They gave her a label
Instead of her son.
She knew in her heart
His soul belonged to no one.
Attempts at reaching him,
Intuitive
Or calculated,
Were clouded
Wistful approximations.

She held on
Hoping
Between them
The rain
And their dreams
The mist might lift. (p. 4)

JOURNAL OF AN ARTIST

ANNE TRUITT'S journal is now published as The Journal of an
Artist *in two parts: "Daybook," from which this excerpt comes,
and "Turn."*

June

New York. The East River surges past the New York Lying-In Hospital. In a dimension entirely different from the densities of steel
and cement lining its progress on east and west, its waters move
deliberately to and from the Atlantic Ocean.

I stand in a small white room beside a table on which my oldest
child lies. Her belly is a mound of stretched skin, her bellybut-
ton, stem of our common blood stream, is flattened to a disk.
From smears of jelly on her stomach, two thin wires attach her
to a black box. The doctor flicks a switch, and we hear an echo

of the Malabar caves. "The baby's heartbeat is twice as fast as the mother's," the doctor remarks. The heartbeat is as impersonal in its rhythm as the river outside the window. The child's life is not as yet marked by human reliance on air. I am struck by a note of intent in the sound, as if I were listening to secret wisdom.

Alexandra and I leave the hospital and walk up and down the streets of New York, happily stopping here and there to buy this or that for the baby. We walk arm in arm, close together—but not as close as my daughter is with her child.

Washington, D.C. Linked only the way yesterday is linked to the morning that rises around me as I write here in my studio, my life led to here, as hers is now leading to her child's. Behind me Portal, a slim column, nine feet of pale, pale grays articulated just off white, looms in its packing. It is ready for shipment to Yaddo, where I will soon be going and where I will finish it. By analogy, I will then cut its umbilical cord and it will fall into place behind First and Queen's Heritage, Landfall, Lea, Hardcastle, and the other sculptures I have made, all synapses through which its life will have come into being.

I comfort myself with this construction, which has risen from my years as an artist, this fact of a continuing succession in my work that offsets a surprisingly bitter impression of having been cast aside. I am disoriented. My motherhood has been, I realize, central to my life as a stove is central to a household in the freeze of winter. I feel chilled. My sculptures are not my children. The construction of an analogy in no sense renders them alive. And I am accustomed to sustaining the effort of my work by offsetting it with the lovely affections of family life.

My mother was dead by the time I had my children. I have been moving for some months now, since the brilliantly sunny morning when we learned that Alexandra was pregnant, into uncharted territory. It so happened that Alexandra and I were alone on that day. We hugged one another in celebration and then came out here to the studio. I worked for a while, painting one light coat of color after another on a column. Alexandra sat on the studio step. We talked. We were quiet. Somehow, quite without emphasis, a new life joined ours.

Now Alexandra and her husband, Richard, have moved through a series of decisions to their present position. They wait in their white-painted, neat apartment for their baby. The crib and the tiny shirts and the pretty cotton blankets are ready. They wait, lovingly, for they know not what.

I know what. I look back over telescoped years. I am waiting for Alexandra's birth, and for Mary's, and for Sam's. I think of vaporizers and suddenly peaked temperatures, of fretful days and long, long hours in parks and of happinesses unexpected and unpredictable. Of prides and disappointments, of angers and joys, of calls on endurance that had to be invented as events demanded it. And of pain, the inevitable pain that marks the mother, peaking into a watershed that cuts off forever the playing fields of childhood. I weep for Alexandra's travail. I brace myself to meet, once again, the knowledge that I cannot take the suffering of my children on myself. That is the essence of motherhood. *Stabat mater:* Mothers can only stand.

My own aspirations fall into a new place. Once again, as at my mother's death, I feel my own mortality, but in my grandchild's birth transmuted into a kind of colorless immortality. Colorless in that it seems to bear no relation to the spirit. I am startled by this fact of the transmission of genes, struck for the first time that matter proliferates from generation to generation without regard for the personalities of the people involved. This new baby already has unimaginably innumerable ova or spermatozoa, some unknowable combination of Alexandra and Richard, of my husband and me, of Richard's parents, of unknown earth-bound forebears. Depersonalized, we live on.

Now, I ask myself, what of the artist who has worked for so long? The steps up and down ladders, the wakings and the goings to sleep with my mind swinging with color, height, breadth, depth? I have only a modest answer: Certainly it does not become less real; certainly it continues. The scale, however, has in some critical way changed. A subtle crack between myself as artist and myself as human being worries me.

I find this situation humbling. I belong to this linked passage of life as unimportantly as the earthworm whose natural functions loosen the earth so that seeds can root easily.

The central emotional fact of my present state of mind— Alexandra's baby is due in about a week now—is not amenable to psychological ratiocination. Lodged like a dark bolus in my midriff is the certain knowledge that my daughter is going to suffer pain. She has never been in pain; she has never even really been sick. Her intact delicacy is like that of an apple blossom. She will be torn.

I turn for relief, for comfort, to my work. . . . (pp. 171–174)

————

Alexandra and Richard have a son. They all three did well. "Incredible" was Alexandra's adjective when she spoke to me on the telephone after the birth. "The baby was crying," she said, and in her voice I caught the unmistakable quiver of motherhood. Reassured, she handed the telephone to Richard and prepared to sleep. She is satisfied with herself; it was a job and she did it well. No fuss and feathers. Richard's voice had the same note of parental responsibility.

They now have a hostage to fortune. Never again will they lean on a window sill as they did yesterday afternoon watching boats on a sunny river, so wholly at their own command. Their son, yesterday in them, is now beyond them. Born, he cannot be protected, and they will never again be carefree. (p. 175)

I STAND HERE IRONING

TILLIE OLSEN wrote short stories during the 1950s about the realities of women's lives that became feminist classics in the following decades. Her story, "Tell Me A Riddle," won the O'Henry Award as the best short story of 1961. Another is excerpted here.

She was a beautiful baby. She blew shining bubbles of sound. She loved motion, loved light, loved color, and music and textures.

She would lie on the floor in her blue overalls patting the surface so hard in ecstasy her hands and feet would blur. She was a miracle to me. (p. 75)

CHILDHOOD

ROBERT LOUIS STEVENSON (1850–1894) achieved both fame and fortune in his brief life. Born in Scotland, he became a lawyer but soon turned to writing adventure stories. Treasure Island *was his first success;* Dr. Jekyll and Mr. Hyde *is considered by many to be his finest work.* The Child's Garden of Verses *remains a beloved children's classic a century after his death. Two poems from that collection follow.*

TO ALISON CUNNINGHAM FROM HER BOY

For the long nights you lay awake:
And watched for my unworthy sake:
For your most comfortable hand
That led me through the uneven land:
For all the story-books you read:
For all the pains you comforted:
For all you pitied, all you bore,
In sad and happy days of yore:
My second Mother, my first Wife,
The angel of my infant life—
From the sick child, now well and old,
Take, nurse, the little book you hold!

And grant it, Heaven, that all who read
May find as dear a nurse at need,
And every child who lists my rhyme,
In the bright fireside nursery clime,
May hear it in as kind a voice
As made my childish days rejoice!

LAND OF COUNTERPANE

When I was sick and lay a-bed,
I had two pillows at my head,

And all my toys beside me lay
To keep me happy all the day.

And sometimes for an hour or so
I watched my leaden soldiers go,
With different uniforms and drills,
Among the bed-clothes, through the hills;

And sometimes sent my ships in fleets
All up and down among the sheets;
Or brought my trees and houses out,
And planted cities all about.

I was the giant great and still
That sits upon the pillow-hill,
And sees before him, dale and plain,
The pleasant land of counterpane. (p. 19)

CHRISTOPHER PIRTLE, AGE 5

CHRISTOPHER PIRTLE's poem is included in Richard Lewis's Journeys: Prose by Children of the English-Speaking World.

I'm not sad. I'm just frowning a very little bit.
That's at the very back. Sad is further up, and
moaning, and being dead is at the very front. I'm
at the back. (p. 157)

FAMILIES

FAMILY ALBUM

ANNE MORROW LINDBERGH is one of America's foremost authors, with many books, poems, and essays on all aspects of life and living. She and her husband, Charles Lindbergh, famous aviator who first crossed the Atlantic alone, suffered the loss of their first-born child when he was kidnapped and murdered. This poem appeared in The Unicorn and Other Poems: 1935–1955.

(On a photograph of my father and mother just married)

My parents, my children:
Who are you, standing there
In an old photograph—young married pair
I never saw before, yet see again?
You pose somewhat sedately side by side,
In your small yard off the suburban road.
He stretches a little in young manhood's pride
Broadening his shoulders for the longed-for load,
The wife he has won, a home his own;
His growing powers hidden as spring, unknown,
But surging in him toward their certain birth,
Explosive as dandelions in the earth.

She leans upon his arm, as if to hide
A strength perhaps too forward for a bride,
Feminine in her bustle and long skirt;
She looks demure, with just a touch of flirt
In archly tilted head and squinting smile
At the photographer, she watches while
Pretending to be girl, although so strong,
Playing the role of wife ("Here I belong!"),
Anticipating mother, with man for child,
Amused at all her roles, unreconciled.

And I who gaze at you and recognize
The budding gestures that were soon to be
My cradle and my home, my trees, my skies,
I am your child, staring at you with eyes
Of love and grief for parents who have died;
But also with omniscience born of time,
Seeing your unlined faces, dreams untried,
Your tentativeness and your brave attack,
I am no longer daughter gazing back;
I am your mother, watching far ahead,
Seeing events so clearly now they're gone
And both of you are dead, and I alone,
And in my own life now already past
That garden in the grass where you two stand.

I long to comfort you for all you two
In time to come must meet and suffer through,
To answer with a hindsight-given truth
The questions in those wondering eyes of youth.
I long to tell you, starting on your quest,
"You'll do it all, you know, you'll meet the test."

Mother compassionate and child bereft
I am; the past and present, wisdom and innocence,
Fused by one flicker of a camera lens
Some stranger snapped in laughter as he left
More than a half a century ago—
My children, my parents. (pp. 79–81)

MOTHER'S DAY

*JOHN COWAN was ordained in 1961 and served as a parish priest,
teacher, and retreat master before leaving to marry and enter
the corporate world. A resident of Minnesota, he is now a consultant, the author of several books, publisher of a newsletter, and
an inveterate sailor. This selection appears in his 1992 book,*
Small Decencies.

One day I was bored and vaguely remembered that a program
was being offered at the Catholic Youth Center that I might even
have signed up for. Knowing that my roman collar opened most
doors, certainly most church doors, I did not hesitate to test my
welcome. By God, I had signed up! I and thirty others were
seated to hear two Episcopal priests address us on "New Models
of Ministry."

As I remember, it was not bad. They did not talk a lot. We played
some nonverbal games and did a little role playing, and one of
them gave a short presentation. It was pleasant and mildly instructive. They mentioned that they were experimenting with a
new-style human-relations workshop and handed out information
on how to attend. Wanting an interesting break in the tedium of
summer, I signed up. I gave it little further thought until the day a

couple of months later when I arrived for a four-day creative risk-taking workshop at the Hudson House in Hudson, Wisconsin.

There is no way to ease into describing this. Most people there found it an emotionally challenging experience. Many tears were shed, many feelings voiced, many hard truths passed on. At one point somebody, in an excess of frustration, put his fist through a wall (not a very sturdy wall, but a wall nevertheless). These were the reactions of normal people.

I was not normal. I had never checked into a motel before. I had never been outside the society of my own church. I had been educated since age thirteen in a monastic male environment. For years my interaction with people had been dampened by the respect thought due a man of the cloth. Here I was, sitting on the floor, in mixed company, trying to articulate my own feelings and hearing how others felt about me—not all of it good! If normal people experienced the workshop as earthshaking, you can imagine my emotional state. I spent my days in semishock and my nights trying to fit this experience into everything else I had learned about life.

At the close of the workshop nearly everyone hugged one another as did I, but with an absence of fervor. Something was vaguely wrong. I liked these folks, but—? I was halfway home when it struck me. I was expressing love and caring for all these people, and I had never told my mother I loved her.

I must do that sometime, I thought on the way home. Perhaps I'll call her when I get to the rectory; after all, I have been gone for four days and there is work to be done. A few miles later I decided I'd call her that day, and after a few more miles, that I would call her and ask her if I could stop by. And by the time I entered the city limits, I decided maybe I'd just drive over to her house *right away*. Driven by my feelings, I rushed through the door in tears. We sat on the sofa and wept before I even began to speak. I told her I loved her. Two years after my mother died, my sister told me that that day was one of the high points in my mother's life. As well it should be. It was a turning point in mine.

For those of us who rush through life trying to do something useful that other people will pay for, it seems to me wise not to forget to touch a few of the critical human bases. I have closed a few sales in my life, and collected a few bonuses, and have been promoted, and I enjoyed and savored every one of these events. But while I know they happened, I only dimly remember them. On the other hand, I could describe to you the angle of the sun, the tilt of the blinds, and the color of her dress the day I told my mother I loved her. (pp. 99–101)

OCTOBER

ANNE TRUITT, in this selection, describes a two-month period during which the author coped with her son's accident and the meanings of creation and relationship. It has been greatly abridged as presented here.

On the night of October 5th the telephone rang. Already in bed, I reached for it rather absentmindedly. A deliberate, female voice asked if this were Mrs. Anne Truitt. I said, "Yes." "This is Suburban Hospital. Your son has been in an automobile accident." I saw Sam's white shirttails hanging down the back of his jeans as, just a short time ago, he had turned out the door with, "See you later, Mom," over his shoulder, off with a friend to pick up another for a study session at his school. The upper reaches of my head seemed to elongate. Some inner silence opened. My body began to hum with energy. . . . (p. 186)

A neurosurgeon had seen Sam; an orthopedic surgeon had been called; a trauma specialist had already checked him and given orders. A nurse hovered over him. He was due for X-rays. There was no way to check his injuries until that was done. By the time he went off for the X-rays, the other parents and the headmaster of his school had arrived. The plastic surgeon got to work on one of the boys and stayed to sew up Sam's neck and face. By that time he had been X-rayed. A broken pelvis, internal injuries of un-known extent. The neurosurgeon stayed on call. The trauma spe-cialist returned to look at him. No water, no medication for pain because of the possibility of brain damage or of extensive inter-nal injuries that might need an immediate operation. Sam twisted and turned with pain, I was relieved to see. No paralysis. And no whining. He endured well. He was going to be able to walk; no spinal injury as far as they could tell. . . . (pp. 188–189)

Sam was hurt three weeks ago today. It is as if the ocean floor of my being had erupted and all my waters had been disturbed. We all felt the quake, but in the other members of the family the waves have subsided. Sam himself is crutching around cheerfully. A piece of glass in his neck is something added; a tooth is some-thing missing. My mind is moving in that loose way these days, as if unhinged: "Something old, something new," silly catch phrases. I feel aquiver. My span of attention is short. I try to think but keep circling back to the fact that Sam's body, once perfectly whole, is now broken. His pelvis is mending but will be forever crooked; not enough to show but out of alignment. Like my sculptures, he went out into the world and got broken, but I cannot mend him as I can them. I move uneasily in a new dimension of helplessness. The artist is no comfort to the mother here. I glance out of the kitchen window at my studio as if it were invisible.

November

Sam is recovering. For the past twenty-four hours I have felt him mending, his proportions coming into proper order. Some shrill, carking note that has been jangling us both stopped last night. The relief is as keen as that felt when a wailing baby is put to the breast. My proportions, too, are slipping back into place, and I am on an even keel again for the first time since the accident. The uter-ine cramps that have been intermittent since October 5th are de-creasing, have stopped almost entirely. This reaction strikes me as bizarre, but, since it is true, I have necessarily to recognize its reality. It is as if I had to take Sam back into the uterus to protect him, to reestablish the placental connection in order to nourish him through his crisis. Perhaps because of this primitive reaction, his recovery is marked by an increasing independence for both of us, a feeling of health and ease as if, in some mysterious way, he had accomplished his second birth, into adulthood, by means of this violent accident. (pp. 191–192)

AGING

From THE VETERAN

DOROTHY PARKER (1893–1967), American author and critic of books and theater for The New Yorker, *is remembered for her acerbic wit and economy of expression. The only woman member of the Algonquin Round Table, she wrote short stories, the most famous of which is "Big Blonde," and satirical poems.*

When I was young and bold and strong,
Oh, right was right, and wrong was wrong!
My plume on high, my flag unfurled,
I rode away to right the world.
"Come out, you dogs, and fight!" said I,
And wept there was but once to die.

But I am old; and good and bad
Are woven in a crazy plaid.

COURAGE

ANNE SEXTON (1928–1974), one of America's most important modern poets, received the Pulitzer Prize for poetry in 1974 for Live or Die. *The poem "Courage" comes from her eighth book of poems,* The Awful Rowing Toward God.

It is in the small things we see it.
The child's first step,
as awesome as an earthquake.

The first time you rode a bike,
wallowing up the sidewalk.
The first spanking when your heart
went on a journey all alone.
When they called you crybaby
or poor or fatty or crazy
and made you into an alien,
you drank their acid
and concealed it.

Later,
if you faced the death of bombs and bullets
you did not do it with a banner,
you did it with only a hat to
cover your heart.
You did not fondle the weakness inside you
though it was there.
Your courage was a small coal
that you kept swallowing.
If your buddy saved you
and died himself in so doing,
then his courage was not courage,
it was love; love as simple as shaving soap.

Later,
if you have endured a great despair,
then you did it alone,
getting a transfusion from the fire,
picking the scabs off your heart,
then wringing it out like a sock.
Next, my kinsman, you powdered your sorrow,
you gave it a back rub
and then you covered it with a blanket
and after it had slept a while
it woke to the wings of the roses
and was transformed.

Later,
when you face old age and its natural conclusion
your courage will still be shown in the little ways,

each spring will be a sword you'll sharpen,
those you love will live in a fever of love,
and you'll bargain with the calendar
and at the last moment
when death opens the back door
you'll put on your carpet slippers
and stride out. (pp. 425–426)

BODIES OF KNOWLEDGE

*GLORIA STEINEM, pioneering feminist, leader of the women's move-
ment, and founder of* Ms. *magazine, has written many articles
and editorials. Her most recent book is* Revolution from Within:
A Book of Self-Esteem, *from which this excerpt is taken. ROBIN
MORGAN, whose poem she quotes, is a feminist poet and author,
and editor of* Ms. *magazine. Her books include* Sisterhood is
Global *and* Upstairs in the Garden, *a collection of poems.*

. . . I celebrated my fiftieth birthday in a very public way by
turning it into a feminist benefit (which I hope my funeral will
also be), and tried to offer some encouragement to other women
facing the double standard of aging by getting as far out of the
age closet as possible. Of course, I continued to hear "fifty" as old
when applied to other people and had consciously and constantly
to revise my own assumptions. Though I began making an effort
to use time better and to understand that my life wasn't going to
go on forever—that is, to use turning fifty to good purposes—my
heart wasn't in it. In fact, I didn't revise one single thing about my
living habits: no exercise except running through airports; no
change in my sugar-addicted habits; no admission that this long
plateau in the middle of my life might be leading into new terrain.
In a way, I felt I *couldn't* acknowledge limitations or any of the
weaknesses to which flesh is heir; the everyday emergencies of a
magazine and a movement were all-consuming, and I didn't think
I could stop swimming in midstream. But to a larger degree, I just
didn't know how. I didn't have a model of how to get from here to
there; from where I was to seventy, eighty, and hopefully beyond.
I needed a model not of *being old,* but of *aging.*

Thanks to good genes, I got away with all this defiance for quite a while—which may be exactly why I needed the word *cancer* to come into my life. Nothing less than such a bodily warning would have made me think about the way I was living. Sleeplessness and endless stress, a quart of ice-cream at a time, and my lifetime rule of no exercise: I was so unaccustomed to listening to any kind of messages from within that I'd ceased to be able to hear even a whisper from that internal voice that must ultimately be our guide. In fact, I had no patience at all with anyone who suggested it was there to be listened to.

Cancer changed that. It gave me a much-needed warning, and it taught me something else: it was not death I had been defying. On the contrary, when I got this totally unexpected diagnosis, my first thought was a bemused, "So this is how it's all going to end." My second was, "I've had a wonderful life." Such acceptance may sound odd, but I felt those words in every last cell of my being. It was a moment I won't forget.

Eventually, that diagnosis and my reaction to it made me realize that I'd been worrying about aging; that my denial and defiance were related to giving up a way of being, not ceasing to be. Though I would have decried all the actresses, athletes, and other worshipers of youth who were unable to imagine a changed future—a few of whom have even chosen death *over* aging—I had been falling into the same trap.

For this health warning—plus the dawning of an understanding that to fear aging is really to fear a new stage of life—I was fortunate to pay only a small price. Thanks to the impact of the women's health movement on at least some of the health-care system, my treatment consisted of a Novocain shot and a biopsy at a women's clinic, while I watched an infinitesimal lump being removed in what turned out to be its entirety—rather like taking out an oddly placed splinter. Since the mammogram had shown nothing—15 percent show false negatives, which is another reason for self-examination—the diagnosis of malignancy was a shock. But what came after was not nearly as difficult as what many women have faced. First, there was a lymph-node sampling that did require going into a hospital, but didn't interfere with going dancing the evening I got out. Since the sampling was negative, the rest of the treatment consisted of six weeks of lying like the Bride of Frankenstein on a metal slab each morning while I got radiation treatments. My self-treatment was much more drastic: doing away with all animal fat in my diet, and getting less stress and more sleep. All this has helped me remain cancer-free for the last five years.

Nonetheless, I was frightened enough by this timely warning to start doing what I needed to do, indeed what I should have been doing all along: listening to what my physical self had to say. Perhaps one of the rewards of aging is a less forgiving body that transmits its warnings faster—not as betrayal, but as wisdom. Cancer makes one listen more carefully, too. I began to seek out a healthier routine, a little introspection, and the time to do my own writing, all of which are reflected in these pages. . . . (pp. 244–246)

In my current stage of aging and listening, I've learned the importance of starting with the body and all its senses. Which is why I go to my body to ask what this new country of aging will be like. . . . (p. 247)

. . . I have a new role model for this adventurous new country I'm now entering. She is a very old, smiling, wrinkled, rosy, beautiful woman, standing in the morning light of a park in Beijing. Her snow-white hair is just visible under a jaunty lavender babushka. Jan Phillips, who took her photograph, says she was belting out a Chinese opera to the sky, stopped for a moment to smile at the camera, and then went on singing. Now, she smiles at me every morning from my mantel.

I love this woman. I like to think that, walking on the path ahead of me, she looks a lot like my future self.

This is the wisdom: If we bless our bodies, they will bless us. In Robin Morgan's poem, "Network of the Imaginary Mother," there is her own version of a pagan prayer: (p. 248)

Blessed be my brain
    that I may conceive of my own power
Blessed be my breast
    that I may give sustenance to those I love.
Blessed be my womb
    that I may create what I choose to create.
Blessed be my knees
    that I may bend so as not to break.
Blessed be my feet
    that I may walk in the path of my highest will.

(from *Upstairs in the Garden,* 1990)

RITES OF ANCIENT RIPENING

Writer and Poet

MERIDEL LESUEUR, 93, has been a writer most of her life, and continues to write daily, living in Wisconsin.

I am luminous with age
In my lap I hold the valley
I see on the horizon what has been taken . . .
In my breast I hold the middle valley . . .
Like corn I cry in the last sunset . . .

    My bones shine in fever
Smoked with the fires of age.

KOROUA

DIANA GRANT-MACKIE, a New Zealand nurse, wrote this poem for a Maori teacher who had a heart condition and would not rest. She describes him:

He was from a tribe called "the children of the mist," hence the reference in the last verse. He also had great standing among all teachers of his era and taught me a great deal about cross-cultural relationships when I visited his school. He has since

*died but, as a teacher of all those who came in contact with
him, he left many people influenced by his life.*

E hoki mai, koroua, return to your youth.
To the pure and simple delight of being alive,
Of standing tall and seeing the world all at once
In one single glance, it is all there.
You have to lean back to do that.

Have you seen the mynah lately
Filling its stomach up in the loquat tree?
And the bright green of the new leaves of Spring
Looking really good with the blue of the sky?
You have to lean back to do that.

Remember the feel of flying over the grass
At sports training in the peak of the season?
The clouds do that now in the wind,
And the long grass too, in bursts of speed.
You have to lean back to feel that.

Hear the noise of the children on the windy days
As they race with the wind and struggle against it.
You run too with your heart and your mind
And fill yourself with their cries of discovery.
You have to lean back to hear that.

Let the seas come back to your eyes, koroua,
With the knowledge down deep but the surface asparkle.
Let the mist of your life drift over the land
And nourish the young with your gift of experience.
You can lean back and do that.

[hoki mai, pronounced hoh-kee my, means "return";
koroua, pronounced cor-oh-wah, means "old man"]

WARNING

*JENNY JOSEPH, respected English poet and writer, has published
four poetry collections and six children's books. Her latest book*

of prose and verse, Persephone, *won the James Tait Memorial Book Prize for fiction in 1986. "When I Am An Old Woman I Shall Wear Purple" serves as the title for a collection of poems about women and aging edited by Sandra Martz (1987).*

When I am an old woman I shall wear purple
With a red hat which doesn't go, and doesn't suit me.
And I shall spend my pension on brandy and summer
    gloves
And satin sandals, and say we've no money for butter.
I shall sit down on the pavement when I'm tired
And gobble up samples in shops and press alarm bells
And run my stick along the public railings
And make up for the sobriety of my youth.
I shall go out in my slippers in the rain
And pick the flowers in other people's gardens
And learn to spit.

You can wear terrible shirts and grow more fat
And eat three pounds of sausages at a go
Or only bread and pickle for a week
And hoard pens and pencils and beermats and things
    in boxes.

But now we must have clothes that keep us dry
And pay our rent and not swear in the street
And set a good example for the children.
We must have friends to dinner and read the papers.

But maybe I ought to practise a little now?
So people who know me are not too shocked and
    surprised
When suddenly I am old, and start to wear purple.

I Grow Old Before My Time

T. S. Eliot (1888–1965), American-born poet and literary critic, won the Nobel Prize for Literature in 1948. His best-known works include The Wasteland *and* The Love Song of J. Alfred Prufrock, *excerpted here.*

I grow old . . . I grow old . . .
I shall wear the bottoms of my trousers rolled.
  Shall I part my hair behind? Do I dare to eat a
peach?
I shall wear white flannel trousers, and walk upon
the beach.
I have heard the mermaids singing, each to each.
I do not think that they will sing to me.

THE AUTUMN OF MY LIFE

POLLY FRANCIS (1884–1978), fashion illustrator and photographer, wrote a series of articles on old age when she was between the ages of ninety-one and ninety-four. This, the first article, was printed in the Congressional Record of April 22, 1975.

What a baffling thing old age is! It doesn't bring the peace we were led to expect. I find it hard to drift with the stream; all along the way there are problems which obstruct the smooth flow of life. The area which lies between the "here" and the "hereafter" is a difficult passage to travel. One must make the journey to fully understand it.

The pattern of life today is such that, at a certain point, it seems desirable that we should leave the main stream and be channeled into a small tributary where the flow is at a gentler speed. But even here there are obstacles.

While our responsibilities lessen, our limitations and frustrations increase—and certain humiliations can be painful.

Our young folk want to be kind to us, I'm sure. But they don't know what we want and they don't know how we feel. What I crave is withheld, so I go winnowing my way around problems and trying to avoid a head-on crash.

The young people may think that we are unreasoningly demanding. It seems to them that all our needs are met. We are comfortably housed, well fed, protected from hazards, provided with companionship and divertissements. What else do we need?

Our greatest need is not met. It is one that we never outgrow. It is the need to feel cherished by someone—to know that there is a place where we "belong." This is something that no retirement home, nursing home or hospital can provide. These institutions are staffed by dedicated people, but it is not their function to soothe our yearning hearts. The emotional strain would be too heavy.

I've been told that I must not succumb to the facts of my age. But why shouldn't I? I am now in my 91st year and I doubt that my activity, for example, in civic affairs, could restore my spirits to a state of bouncing buoyancy. Lack of physical strength alone keeps me inactive and often silent. I've been called senile. Senility is a convenient peg upon which to hang our nonconformity.

Age creeps up so stealthily that it is often with shock that we become aware of its presence. Perhaps that is why so many of us reach old age utterly unprepared to meet its demands. We may be a bit rebellious about accepting it; I want to cry out that the invisible part of me is not old. I still thrill to the beauties of this world—the dew upon the rose at dawn, the glow reflected by the sun on passing cloud when day is done—but unremitting age goes on.

My interest in the goings-on in the world outside my ever-tightening barriers has not been withdrawn. It is not interest that I have lost, but rather the means of getting around and the physical stamina to sustain me as I go.

It is my task now to build a new life. My renunciations are many. The component parts with which I shall build are sometimes unfamiliar and often unappealing. At first a bleak stretch of nothingness seemed to lie before me; I yearned for my comfortable deep furrow dug by my habits of many years.

In earlier times I didn't look beyond the move of the moment. Each move seemed almost fixed and final. But now all feeling of permanency has slipped away. The thought of where I shall go from here lurks in my consciousness. Will it be to a nursing home, or to a hospital or shall I go directly with no stopovers? Whichever it will be, I shall look upon it with no dread.

My new life is taking shape. The barriers of my little world are closing in on me. I am not sad or discontented—just very tired. If I sit alone at twilight, it is because I need solitude and rest. My solace is my memories, left untouched by the devastating hand of time. Tears, too, help—tears of tenderness; tears of grief have dried away. I do not mourn "good old days." I've had them. I've enjoyed them and my memory will preserve them.

The room in which I spend my days and nights is quietly pleasant and comfortable, with a large window looking out over the tree-tops toward a distance, jagged horizon. It is not merely an enclosure where my few remaining possessions are stored and where I am safe from the common hazards of living alone; it is the setting of a new kind of life to which I am trying to adjust.

A new set of faculties seems to be coming into operation. I seem to be awakening to a larger world of wonderment—to catch little glimpses of the immensity and diversity of creation. More than at any other time in my life, I seem to be aware of the beauties of our spinning planet and the sky above. And now I have the time to enjoy them. I feel that old age sharpens our awareness.

I sit by my window and watch a thing of great beauty die with the setting sun. It is gone forever. Time loses its importance. On a bright, clear day, what a challenge to my imagination is the sight of an azure sky with balls of white fluff tumbling and rolling and gathering and dispersing and endlessly forming fantastic patterns.

In the quiet of the night, a siren sounds. A pang of compassion strikes into my heart. I want to rush to the scene of distress, but how utterly useless I've become. I look out at the red lights blinking reassurance to the night travelers streaking through the sky. What emotions these planes carry!

My window has become a showcase of ever-changing wonderment. The objects in my room take on different aspects with the shifting sun. Like actors on a stage, each thing has its moment in the limelight.

I pick up a much-read book and in it I find new delights. I watch an ant persistently toiling with a tiny bit of something and I realize

that a spark of the Great Universal Will keeps it going undespair-
ingly. I look at a cobweb and wonder at the spider's weaving skill
and engineering know-how.

The telephone rings. My heart leaps. For a few minutes I listen to
a beloved voice. Distance is wiped away. I am no longer on alien
ground. I am where I "belong."

When my courage turns limp, I ponder my past. I try to find a
yardstick with which to measure the merit of a life. I become so
confused that I cannot tell right from wrong. They come so close
together and dance so fast from side to side that I am unable to
grasp them firmly. And that is where faith comes in. We cannot
know; we can only believe.

Old age is not all pain and limitations. It holds its own joys and
satisfactions. The time has come when musing replaces activities—when the sleepless hours are filled from the harvest of a
well-stored mind. Even though our means are scant, we know that
our material needs will, somehow, be met. But an impoverished
soul is a saddening thing.

One of my joys is the spontaneous kindness of people everywhere—in the home where I live, in the shops, in the street—
wherever my faltering step is noticed. It fills me with a warm glow.
The quickness of the young boys and girls and the ease and non-
chalance with which they offer help give me the feeling that they
are trying to minimize my helplessness. I admire them without
reservation.

The common expression, "so-and-so is failing," is tossed around
too freely. In aging we gain as well as lose. The autumn of human
life, like the autumn of nature, can bring richness of beauty. It's a
time when our spiritual forces seem to expand. A life of the heart
and of the mind takes over while our physical force ebbs away.

THE SAILING INSTRUCTOR

JOHN COWAN, author of the earlier selection, Mother's Day.

My mother went to a rest home in her early seventies. She suffered from osteoporosis, and over the last few years she had been

gradually losing control over her body. She doubled over, had trouble lifting her head, could not raise her voice. As she was pushed down the street in a wheelchair, her head tended to precede the chair, looking not unlike the figurehead on the bow of a ship.

I came up to the fourth floor to see her one day and the nurse at the station said to me, with a smile, "Have your mother tell you how she called the cops on us."

There was nothing wrong with Ruth's mind up to this point. But as I hurried down the hall I wondered if she had begun slipping. She told me the story in the barely audible voice that went with the badly crippled body.

"I woke this morning needing to go to the bathroom. The bell to call the nurses was behind me, pinned to the bed. I can no longer roll over without help. I tried. I tried calling out, but nobody could hear me. I am not soiling my bed if I can help it. The phone was reachable. I dialed 911 and told them to call the nursing home and tell them that the woman in 409 needs to go to the bathroom. Let me tell you, I got quick service."

Way to go, Mom. (p. 117)

CREATIVITY AND LONGEVITY

NORMAN COUSINS

Some observations about Pablo Casals.

I met him for the first time at his home in Puerto Rico just a few weeks before his ninetieth birthday. I was fascinated by his daily routine. At 8 A.M. his lovely young wife Marta would help him to start the day. His various infirmities made it difficult for him to dress himself. Judging from his difficulty in walking and from the way he held his arms, I guessed he was suffering from rheumatoid arthritis. His emphysema was evident in his labored breathing. He came into the living room on Marta's arm. He was badly stooped. His head was pitched forward and he walked with a shuffle. His hands were swollen and his fingers were clenched.

Even before going to the breakfast table, Don Pablo went to the piano—which, I learned, was a daily ritual. He arranged himself with some difficulty on the piano bench, then with discernible effort raised his swollen and clenched fingers above the keyboard.

I was not prepared for the miracle that was about to happen. The fingers slowly unlocked and reached toward the keys like the buds of a plant toward the sunlight. His back straightened. He seemed to breathe more freely. Now his fingers settled on the keys. Then came the opening bars of Bach's *Wohltemperierte Klavier,* played with great sensitivity and control. I had forgotten that Don Pablo had achieved proficiency on several musical instruments before he took up the cello. He hummed as he played, then said that Bach spoke to him here—and he placed his hand over his heart.

Then he plunged into a Brahms concerto and his fingers, now agile and powerful, raced across the keyboard with dazzling speed. His entire body seemed fused with the music; it was no longer stiff and shrunken but supple and graceful and completely freed of its arthritic coils.

Having finished the piece, he stood up by himself, far straighter and taller than when he had come into the room. He walked to the breakfast table with no trace of a shuffle, ate heartily, talked animatedly, finished the meal, then went for a walk on the beach. . . . (pp. 72–73)

. . . A man almost ninety, beset with the infirmities of old age, was able to cast off his afflictions, at least temporarily, because he knew he had something of overriding importance to do. There was no mystery about the way it worked, for it happened every day. Creativity for Pablo Casals was the source of his own cortisone. It is doubtful whether any antiinflammatory medication he would have taken would have been as powerful or as safe as the substances produced by the interaction of his mind and body. (p. 74)

DO NOT GO GENTLE INTO THAT GOOD NIGHT

DYLAN MARLAIS THOMAS (1914–1953), Welsh poet and bard, published his first collection, Eighteen Poems, *at age 20. His major works such as "Under Milk Wood" and "A Child's Christmas in Wales" were written for radio performance. However, "Do Not Go Gentle into That Good Night" remains his best known poem.*

Do not go gentle into that good night,
Old age should burn and rave at close of day;
Rage, rage against the dying of the light.

Though wise men at their end know dark is right,
Because their words had forked no lightning they
Do not go gentle into that good night.

Good men, the last wave by, crying how bright
Their frail deeds might have danced in a green bay,
Rage, rage against the dying of the light.

Wild men who caught and sang the sun in flight,
And learn, too late, they grieved it on its way,
Do not go gentle into that good night.

Grave men, near death, who see with blinding sight
Blind eyes could blaze like meteors and be gay,
Rage, rage against the dying of the light.

And you, my father, there on the sad height,
Curse, bless me now with your fierce tears, I pray.
Do not go gentle into that good night.
Rage, rage against the dying of the light. (p. 215)

IX

ON DYING AND GRIEVING

Something has spoken to me in the night, burning the tapers of the waning year, something has spoken in the night, and told me I shall die, I know not where.

Saying: To lose the earth you know, for greater life; to leave the friends you loved, for greater loving; to find a land more kind than home, more large than earth;

Whereon the pillars of this earth are founded, toward which the conscience of the world is tending—a wind is rising, and the rivers flow.

Thomas Wolfe, *You Can't Go Home, Again,* 1940

Since the beginning of time, persons have searched as assid-uously for the meaning of death as for the meaning of life. It is difficult to say who searches harder, those approaching death, those witnessing death, or those left behind. Health professionals cannot escape. They must ease the dying and comfort the living. For the reader, literature is a way of knowing death and grieving and, for the writer, literature is a way of sharing what has been experienced and learned.

* * *

DEATH BE NOT PROUD

*JOHN DONNE (1572–1631), English metaphysical poet and the-
ologian, served as chaplain to James I and dean of St. Paul's
Cathedral. His works include* Divine Poems *(1607).*

Death be not proud, though some have called thee
Mighty and dreadful, for, thou art not so,
For, those, whom thou think'st, thou dost overthrow,
Die not, poor death, nor yet canst thou kill me;
From rest and sleep, which but thy pictures be,
Much pleasure, then from thee, much more must flow,
And soonest our best men with thee do go,
Rest of their bones, and soul's delivery.
Thou art slave to fate, chance, kings, and desperate men,
And dost with poison, war, and sickness dwell,
And poppy, or charms can make us sleep as well,
And better than thy stroke; why swell'st thou then?
One short sleep past, we wake eternally,
And death shall be no more, Death thou shalt die.

HOSPITAL SKETCHES

LOUISA MAY ALCOTT, more from her writings about the Civil War.

My own experiences of this sort began when my first man died.
He had scarcely been removed, when his wife came in. Her eye
went straight to the well-known bed; it was empty; and feeling,
yet not believing the hard truth, she cried out, with a look I never
shall forget:

"Why, where's Emanuel?"

I had never seen her before, did not know her relationship to the
man whom I had only nursed for a day, and was about to tell her
he was gone, when McGee, the tender-hearted Irishman before
mentioned, brushed by me with a cheerful—"It's shifted to a better bed he is, Mrs. Connel. Come out, dear, till I show ye"; and,

taking her gently by the arm, he led her to the matron, who broke the heavy tidings to the wife, and comforted the widow.

Another day, running up to my room for a breath of fresh air and a five minutes' rest after a disagreeable task, I found a stout young woman sitting on my bed, wearing the miserable look which I had learned to know by that time. Seeing her, reminded me that I had heard of some one's dying in the night, and his sister's arriving in the morning. This must be she, I thought. I pitied her with all my heart. What could I say or do? Words always seem impertinent at such times; I did not know the man; the woman was neither interesting in herself nor graceful in her grief; yet, having known a sister's sorrow myself, I could not leave her alone with her trouble in that strange place, without a word. So, feeling heart-sick, home-sick, and not knowing what else to do, I just put my arms about her, and began to cry in a very helpless but hearty way; for, as I seldom indulge in this moist luxury, I like to enjoy it with all my might, when I do.

It so happened I could not have done a better thing; for, though not a word was spoken, each felt the other's sympathy; and, in the silence, our handkerchiefs were more eloquent than words. She soon sobbed herself quiet; and, leaving her on my bed, I went back to work, feeling much refreshed by the shower, though I'd forgotten to rest, and had washed my face instead of my hands. I mention this successful experiment as a receipt proved and approved, for the use of any nurse who may find herself called upon to minister to these wounds of the heart. They will find it more efficacious than cups of tea, smelling-bottles, psalms, or sermons; for a friendly touch and a companionable cry, unite the consolations of all the rest for womankind; and, if genuine, will be found a sovereign cure for the first sharp pang so many suffer in these heavy times. (pp. 92–93)

THE PRINCESS

ALFRED LORD TENNYSON (1809–1892) was a British poet whose many poems reflect Victorian sentiments. Among the best known are "The Charge of the Light Brigade," "Crossing the Bar," *and* "In Memoriam." *Excerpted here is one brief section of his lengthy epic poem,* "The Princess."

Home they brought her warrior dead:
    She nor swooned, nor uttered cry:
All her maidens, watching, said,
    "She must weep or she will die."

Then they praised him, soft and low,
    Called him worthy to be loved,
Truest friend and noblest foe;
    Yet she neither spoke nor moved.

Stole a maiden from her place,
    Lightly to the warrior stept,
Took the face-cloth from the face;
    Yet she neither moved nor wept.

Rose a nurse of ninety years,
    Set his child upon her knee—
Like summer tempest came her tears—
    "Sweet my child, I live for thee." (p. 267)

THERE'S BEEN A DEATH

EMILY DICKINSON

There's been a Death, in the Opposite House,
As lately as Today—
I know it, by the numb look
Such Houses have—alway—

The Neighbors rustle in and out—
The Doctor—drives away—
A Window opens like a Pod—
Abrupt—mechanically—

Somebody flings a Mattress out—
The Children hurry by—

They wonder if it died—on that—
I used to—when a Boy—

The Minister—goes stiffly in—
As if the House were His—
And He owned all the Mourners—now—
And little Boys—besides—

And then the Milliner—and the Man—
Of the Appalling Trade—
To take the measure of the House—

There'll be that Dark Parade—

Of Tassels—and of Coaches—soon—
It's easy as a Sign—
The Intuition of the News—
In just a country Town—

INTERMINABLE LIFE

ISABEL ALLENDE, Chilean journalist, long a resident of Caracas, Venezuela, turned to writing fiction in 1981 and enjoyed instant success with the publication of The House of the Spirits. *The following story is taken from* The Stories of Eva Luna, *1989.*

There are all kinds of stories. Some are born with the telling; their substance is language, and before someone puts them into words they are but a hint of an emotion, a caprice of mind, an image, or an intangible recollection. Others are manifest whole, like an apple, and can be repeated infinitely without risk of altering their meaning. Some are taken from reality and process through inspiration, while others rise up from an instant of inspiration and become real after being told. And then there are secret stories that remain hidden in the shadows of the mind; they are like living organisms, they grow roots and tentacles, they become covered with excrescences and parasites, and with time are transformed into the matter of nightmares. To exorcise the demons of memory, it is sometimes necessary to tell them as a story.

Ana and Roberto Blaum had grown old together. They were so close that over the years they had come to look like brother and sister; they had the same expression of benevolent surprise, the same wrinkles, the same hand gestures, the same lope of the shoulder; they had been shaped by similar habits and desires. For the greater part of their lives they had shared each day, and from having walked so far hand in hand, and having slept so long in each other's arms, they could agree to rendezvous in the same dream. They had never been apart since their meeting a half-century before. At that time, Roberto had been studying medicine, and had already exhibited the passion that rules his life: to purify the world and serve his fellowman. Ana was one of those virginal young girls whose innocence makes everything about her more beautiful. They discovered each other through music. Ana was a violinist in a chamber orchestra and he—who came from a family of virtuosos and himself enjoyed playing the piano—never missed a concert. . . .

. . . Even though the war had delayed his studies, Roberto Blaum's successes had begun early in his career. When another physician might just have begun practicing, Roberto had published several respected articles. His true reputation, however, was the result of his book on the right to a peaceful death. He was not tempted by private practice, except in the case of some friend or neighbor, but preferred to pursue his profession in public hospitals where he could attend a greater number of sick and every day learn something new. Long hours in the wards of terminal patients had instilled in him a great compassion for those fragile bodies chained to life-support machines, with all the torture of their needles and tubes, patients whom science had denied their final dignity under the pretext that they must be kept breathing at any cost. It troubled him not to be able to help such people depart this world but to be forced, instead, to hold them against their will on their deathbeds. On occasion, the suffering imposed on his patients became so intolerable that he could think of nothing else. At night, when he slept, Ana would have to wake him when he cried out. In the refuge of their bed, he would embrace his wife, burying his face in her breasts, despairing.

"Why don't you disconnect the tubes and relieve that poor man's suffering? It is the most merciful thing you can do. He's going to die anyway, sooner or later . . . ."

"I can't do it, Ana. The law is very clear; no one has the right to take another's life, although in my mind, this is a matter of conscience."

"We've been through this before, and every time you suffer the same remorse. No one will know; it will take only a minute or two."

Whether Roberto ever did, only Ana knew. In his view, death, with its ancestral weight of terrors, is merely the abandonment of an unserviceable shell at the time the spirit is reintegrated into the unified energy of the cosmos. The end of life, like birth, is a stage in a voyage, and deserves the compassion we accord to its beginnings. There is absolutely no virtue in prolonging the heartbeat and tremors of a body beyond its natural span, and the physician's labor should be to ease our passing, rather than contribute to the objectionable bureaucracy of death. These decisions, however, should not be left solely to the judgment of professionals or the compassion of family members; the law must establish a set of criteria.

Blaum's proposal evoked an uproar from priests, lawyers, and doctors. Soon the matter transcended scientific circles and spilled over to public debate, sharply dividing opinions. For the first time someone had spoken out on the subject; until then, death had been a taboo topic. One wagered on immortality, with the secret hope of living forever. As long as the discussion was maintained at a philosophical level, Roberto Blaum participated in public forums to argue his thesis, but once the subject became a diversion of the masses, he took refuge in his work, offended by the shamelessness with which his theory was being exploited for commercial purposes. Death took center stage; stripped of all reality, it became *fashionable*.

One element of the press accused Blaum of promoting euthanasia and compared his tenets to those of the Nazis, while another element acclaimed him as a saint. He ignored the tumult and continued his research and work at the hospital. His book was translated into several languages and published in other countries, where it provoked similarly impassioned reactions. His photograph appeared frequently in scientific journals. That year he was offered a Chair in the Medical School, and soon was the professor most sought after by students. There was not an ounce of arrogance in Roberto Blaum nor of the exultant fanaticism of mediums of divine revelation, only the scholar's placid conviction. The greater Roberto's fame, the more reclusive the Blaums' life became. The impact of that brief celebrity startled them, and they admitted fewer and fewer into their intimate circle.

Roberto's theory was forgotten by the public as quickly as it had become faddish. The law was not changed; the problem was not even debated in Congress, but in the academic and scientific worlds Blaum's prestige steadily grew. In the following thirty years, Blaum trained several generations of surgeons, developed new drugs and surgical techniques, and organized a system of mobile consultation facilities—vans, boats, and planes equipped for treating everything from childbirth to epidemics—that formed a network across the nation, bringing help to areas where previously only missionaries had chanced. He obtained numerous prizes, for a decade was Rector of the University, and for two weeks he was Minister of Health—the amount of time necessary to gather evidence of administrative corruption and misappropriation of funds and to present the facts to the President, who had no alternative but to destroy them: he could not shake the foundations of the government merely to please an idealist. Through all that time Blaum continued his research on the dying. He published various articles on the obligation to inform the terminal patient of his true condition, so he would have time to prepare his soul and not be stunned by the surprise of dying, and on respecting suicide and other forms of ending one's own life without undue pain and stridency.

Blaum's name again became a household word when he published his last book, which not only rocked traditional science but evoked an avalanche of hope across the nation. In his long hospital practice Roberto had treated innumerable cancer patients and had observed that while some were defeated by death, others given the same treatment survived. In his book Roberto attempted to demonstrate the relationship between cancer and state of mind: he argued that sorrow and loneliness facilitate the reproduction of the deadly cells, because when a patient is depressed, the body's defense system is weakened; if, on the other hand, he has good reason to live, his organism battles tirelessly against the disease. He reasoned that a cure for cancer, therefore, should not be limited to surgery, chemistry, or medical resources, which address only physical manifestations, but that state of mind must be given prime consideration. In the last chapter he suggested that the best results are to be found among those blessed with a loving partner, or some other source of affection, since love has a beneficial effect unsurpassed by even the most powerful drugs.

The press immediately appreciated the limitless possibilities of this theory and placed words in Blaum's mouth that he had never spoken. If his book on death had caused an uproar, now a second, equally natural aspect of life was to be treated as an innovation. All the virtues of the philosopher's stone were attributed to love; it was claimed that it could cure all ills. Everyone talked about Blaum's book, but very few had read it. The simple proposition that affection can be good for health was perverted according to what each individual wanted to add to or remove from the equation, until Blaum's original idea was lost in a tangle of absurdities that created a colossal confusion in the average mind. There was, naturally, no shortage of swindlers willing to take advantage of all this interest, appropriating love as if it were their personal invention. New esoteric sects proliferated, schools of psychology, courses for beginners, clubs for the lonelyheart, pills for fatal attraction, devastating perfumes, and a multitude of garden-variety diviners who used cards and crystal balls to sell cheap fortunes. As soon as it was discovered that Ana and Roberto Blaum were an amiable old couple who had been together for the best part of their lives and had preserved bodily and mental health *and* the strength of their love, they were lionized as living examples of

Blaum's theory. With the exception of the scientists who analyzed the book to the point of exhaustion, the only people who read it for nonsensationalist purposes were people actually suffering from cancer. For them, however, the hope of a definitive cure became an atrocious joke; in fact, no one could tell them where to find love, how to attain it, even less, how to keep it. Although Blaum's idea was not without logic, in practice it was inapplicable.

Roberto was dismayed by the extent of the publicity, but Ana reminded him of what had happened with the first book and convinced him it was only a question of waiting awhile until the hubbub subsided. Which it did. The Blaums, however, were out of the city when the clamor finally died down. Roberto had already retired from his work at the hospital and university, using the excuse that he was tired and at an age when he wanted to live a more tranquil life. He had not, however, been able to escape his own celebrity; his house was invaded at all hours by potential patients, newspaper reporters, students, professors, and curiosity seekers. Roberto told me he needed quiet to work on another book, and I said I would help him find a peaceful refuge. We found a small house in La Colonia, a strange village set into the side of a tropical mountain, a replica of a nineteenth-century Bavarian village, an architectural oddity of painted wood houses, cuckoo clocks, window boxes filled with geraniums, and Gothic-lettered signs; it was inhabited by a race of blonds with the same Tyrolean clothing and rosy cheeks their great-grandparents had brought with them from the Black Forest. Although La Colonia was already the tourist attraction we know today, Roberto was able to rent a cottage far from the weekend traffic. He and Ana asked me to look after things in the capital; I collected his retirement check, their bills, and the mail. At first I visited them fairly often, but soon I realized they were feigning a rather forced cordiality very different from the warmth of my usual welcome. I knew it was nothing personal; I had no doubts about the trust and affection they felt for me. I simply came to the conclusion they wanted to be alone, and found it easier to communicate with them by letter and telephone.

When Roberto Blaum last called me, I had not seen them for a year. Although I often had long conversations with Ana, I had spoken very little with him. I would tell Ana the latest news, and she would tell me stories from their past, which seemed increasingly vivid for her, as if all those distant memories had become part of the present in the silence that now surrounded her. From time to time she sent me the oatmeal cookies she had always baked for me, and sachets of lavender to perfume my closets. Recently she had sent me tender little gifts: a handkerchief her husband had given her years before, photographs of herself as a girl, an antique brooch. I suppose that the gifts, more than their strange remoteness and the fact that Roberto had avoided speaking of the progress of his book, should have been my clue, but in fact I never suspected what was happening in that little house in the mountains. Later, when I read Ana's diary, I learned that Roberto had not written a single line. All that time he had devoted himself solely to loving his wife, but his love had not been able to alter the course of events.

On weekends, the trip to La Colonia becomes a pilgrimage of overheated cars creeping along with wheels barely turning. On weekdays, however, especially during the rainy season, it is a solitary drive along a route of hairpin curves that knife through peaks between surprising ravines and forests of sugar cane and palm trees. That afternoon, clouds trapped among the hills cloaked the landscape in cotton. The weather had stilled the birds, and the only sound was the slap of the rain against the windshield. As I ascended, the air grew cool, and the storm suspended in the fog felt more like the climate of a different latitude. Suddenly, at a bend in the road, I saw that Germanic-looking village with roofs pitched to support a snow that would never fall. To reach the Blaums' house I had to drive through town, which was apparently deserted at that hour. Their cottage was similar to all the others: dark wood with carved eaves and lace-curtained windows. There was a well-tended flower garden in front of the house, and a small plot of strawberries in the rear. A cold wind was whistling through the trees, but I saw no smoke rising from the chimney. The Blaums' old dog did not move when I called; he raised his head and looked at me without wagging his tail, as if he did not recognize me, but followed when I opened the unlocked door and went inside. It was dark. I felt along the wall for the light switch and turned on the lights. Everything was in order. Fresh eucalyptus branches filled the vases, saturating the air with a sharp, clean scent. I walked through the living room of this rented house in which nothing betrayed the Blaums' presence except the stacks of books and Ana's violin, and I was puzzled that in a year and a half my friends had left no trace of their presence.

I climbed the stairs to the main bedroom, a large room with high ceilings and rustic beams, stained wallpaper and inexpensive furniture in a vaguely provincial style. A lamp on the night table lighted the bed where Ana lay in a blue silk dress and the coral necklace I so often saw her wear. In death she had the same expression of innocence as in the wedding photograph taken long ago, the day the ship's captain had married them seventy miles off the coast, that splendid afternoon when flying fish announced to the refugees that the promised land was near. The dog, who had followed me, curled up in a corner, moaning softly.

On the night table, beside an unfinished embroidery and the diary of Ana's life, I found a note to me from Roberto in which he asked me to look after the dog and to bury his wife and himself in one coffin in the cemetery of that fairy-tale village. They had decided to die together; Ana was terminally ill with cancer and they preferred to travel to the next stage of their lives hand in hand, as they had always done, so that at the fleeting instant in which the spirit disengages, they would not run the risk of losing each other in some warp in the vast universe.

I ran through the house, looking for Roberto. I found him behind the kitchen in the small room he used for a study, seated at a wooden desk, his head in his hands, sobbing. On the desk lay the syringe he had used to inject his wife, now filled with the dose intended for him. I rubbed the nape of his neck; he looked up and stared into my eyes for an endless moment. It seemed clear that he had wanted to prevent Ana's terminal suffering and prepared their farewell so that nothing would alter the serenity of the moment; he had cleaned the house, cut fresh branches for the vases, dressed his wife and combed her hair, and when everything was ready he had given her the injection. Consoling her with the promise that a few minutes later he would be joining her, he had lain beside her and held her until he was certain she was no longer alive. He had refilled the syringe, pushed up his shirtsleeve, and located the vein, but then things had not gone as he planned. That was when he had called me.

"I can't do it, Eva. You're the only one I can ask. Please . . . Help me die."

The death of children has evoked overpowering feeling from which has issued a powerful body of writing. Five such selections are presented here. Literature has proved for these writers a way of searching for meaning in death and dealing with grief, and guilt, and other emotions unleashed through such experiences.

BROKEN SHELL

ANNE MORROW LINDBERGH

> Cease searching for the perfect shell, the whole
> Inviolate form no tooth of time has cracked;
> The alabaster armor still intact
> From sand's erosion and the breaker's roll.
>
> What can we salvage from the ocean's strife
> More lovely than these skeletons that lie
> Like scattered flowers open to the sky,
> Yet not despoiled by their consent to life?
>
> The pattern on creation morning laid,
> By softened lip and hollow, unbetrayed;
> The gutted frame endures, a testament,
> Even in fragment, to that first intent.
>
> Look at this spiral, stripped to polished nerve
> Of growth. Erect as compass in its curve,
> It swings forever to the absolute,
> Crying out beauty like a silver flute. (p. 82)

A MEMORIAL

GORDON LIVINGSTON, a psychiatrist, lives in Maryland. He served as a medical officer in Vietnam in 1968–69 and has written on a variety of subjects for several publications. This letter is part of a longer essay written to his 6-year-old son Lucas at the time of the boy's death from leukemia.

Dear Lucas,

Wherever your spirit is now I'm not sure there's mail delivery so I asked my friend, Paul, to read this to you to explain what has happened to temporarily separate us. You knew about leukemia, that it was a serious disease that we had to try to treat so that we could all go on making each other happy in this world. When the doctors explained that your best chance was to get some of my bone marrow I was glad, because I thought that since you and I were so close in every other way, my marrow would get along fine in your body and would help get rid of the leukemia.

For reasons not even the doctors know, after the transplant, the drugs they were using as well as my cells affected certain parts of you like your skin and liver and kidneys. You fought hard to overcome these problems, took your medicines, and did everything you could to recover. Your Mom and I and Emily stayed with you through all of it, trying to keep you comfortable and help you battle the disease that was making you so sick. Many people, some we didn't even know, wrote us and prayed for your recovery. I never saw anyone fight as hard as you did. You never gave up hope and we talked a lot about all the things you wanted to do when you got well. Everyone who took care of you said you were the bravest and best patient they had ever seen. Sometimes I know you felt terrible and some of the procedures were painful. Through it all we kept loving you and you kept loving us. I couldn't believe that you never got angry at the unfairness of all you had to go through. I know I got angry that this had happened to you. I still am. And sorry, Luke, I'm so sorry.

Finally the disease affected so many different parts of your body that it overwhelmed you and you died. Practically your whole family, all the people who loved you most, were with you at the end, talking to you, holding on to you, loving you. We still love you and always will, even though it breaks our hearts not to be able to show it in the way we did when you were here by touching, hugging, kissing you. We believe that you are in a safe place until, one by one, we can join you. I think I'll be the first to come and it makes me happy to think of being with you again. Until then I hope you can see us and feel how much we miss you.

I don't understand why God chose to separate us now. There's a lot about His ways I don't understand but have to accept. You were like an angel placed in our care for a little while and I am so proud to have been your father. It eases my pain that Emily is with us; her shining spirit is so like yours.

And now we're getting ready to put your body in a pretty place under a tulip poplar tree right next to the church. We do this so we can visit every Sunday or whenever we want to be especially close to all our wonderful memories of you. Meanwhile your spirit roams free and, I believe, watches over us. Already the sadness and anger we feel at your not being alive are changing to good thoughts about all you gave us in your short time on earth. So don't worry about our tears now. They'll turn to smiles after we've had time to heal ourselves, when we remember what a funny happy little boy you were and what a joy it was to love you and be loved by you.

Good-bye, Lukey—for a little while.

Dad. (pp. 28–29)

YOU AND I

YUEH-CHIH CHEN is a clinical nurse specialist from The Republic of China; the poem is from her doctoral dissertation on A Taoist Model for Human Caring: The Lived Experiences and Caring Needs of Mothers with Children Suffering from Cancer in Taiwan, *1988.*

You, my child, were born out of our eager expectation.
Your liveliness, loveliness, and naughtiness won our
    admiration.

I took a mother's pride in having you.
That you brought us a lot of pleasure was true.

All of a sudden you fell into a dark valley.
Monsters were waiting to seize you as their prey.
You and I had no peaceful days.
Our pleasant time became memories of yesterday.

I tried to create a better environment for you.
I anxiously sought ways to save you.
I prayed to Goddess to protect you,
    to get you out of the valley and see the beautiful
    rainbow.

In the deadly valley, the monster aimed at you.
Under its sway you got weaker and weaker.
I saw you fight in agony and might lose the day.
I felt guilty for not helping you win the battle.

Now my child, you are losing the battle inch by inch.
My emotions are going down and down.
But I tell you the hope is there.
I encourage you to fight to see the rainbow again.

But your life these days may be in vain.
I pray to Buddha to take you away
    to a secure and beautiful paradise
    or to strengthen you and save you.

No matter where Buddha takes you along,
Our pleasant time will live in memory long.
You will still always be my lively and lovely child
    and I will still forever be your loving mother.

ELEGY TO MY SON

STEINUNN EYJOLFSDOTTIR is an Icelandic author of poems, short stories, children's stories, and articles. These two poems, numbered and nameless, were among a series written following her son's death in a 1985 road accident.

III

When do mother and child
first meet?
It is so strange—
but the thought always recurs
of first having met you in a graveyard.
I was looking for your brother's resting place
in darkness
and wind
and rain
among uncovered graves.
I was alone
and the cold
pierced through my bones.
Then a bright and glad mind
touched mine
and I stretched my hands
out into darkness
and said:
Come to me Dagur.
For I always knew your name
would be Dagur—Day.

———

When does a mother's dream become a real child?
Has this question ever been answered?

IX

I don't know why
your life was so short.
But I do know
that it was infinitely precious
as all lives are.
No boy, no girl
should ever
anywhere
play with life.

Far too much is at stake.
Even a tiny spark of life,
a life with little hope
is like a light
in the great white
cluster of stars
far away and endless

—

Let me tell them that
from you.

One nurse has expressed through poetry her personal grief and moral outrage at the needless deaths of multitudes of women in childbirth in many countries of the world.

Maternal Mortality

Marie-Therese Feuerstein presented this unpublished poem at an international medical assembly in Toronto, Canada, in August 1991.

People don't really understand
How women die in childbirth
The details
Are almost
Unimaginable
The living foetus
Striving for life
Fighting to be born.
The life-going sanctuary
Of the uterus
Becomes the prison,
The tomb.

Or the mother,
Weak from the pain
Of delivery

Finds nothing
Seems able to quell
The gushing of her blood.
There are no more cloths
To absorb the flow,
And only two more hours
To her life.

If we cannot improve
The quality of women's lives
At least improve
The quality of their deaths. . .

How can we "sell"
Maternal mortality?
This human tragedy
is not available
On video.
Anyway
It is a "taboo" subject
Linked
With human sexuality
Which is already
A taboo subject.

Unfortunately,
No-one has interviewed
The dying woman.
We don't know
What she would have to say
To us.
Perhaps
Someone should interview
The children
Whose mothers have died.
They may well wonder
Why their mothers
Had to be pregnant again
In the first place.

It is difficult to sell
A commodity
That is too common.
Anyway, dying is a familiar occupation.
"Why should we
Get excited about maternal deaths
There are so many other kinds. . . !"

Perhaps we have to sell
Maternal mortality
More as a "fin-de-siecle"
Phenomenon.
The question is,
Does maternal mortality matter?

If it doesn't,
Perhaps we should approach with caution
Entry into a century
Where women will go on dying
In increasing numbers
And where . . .
It still won't matter.

Deathbed vigils are awash with emotion for the loved ones. Role playing, reminiscences, personal vulnerability are exposed in literature about such experiences. Two such pieces follow.

A Very Easy Death

Simone de Beauvoir (1908–1986) was a French feminist and existentialist whose works include The Second Sex *(1949) and* The Coming of Age *(1970), cultural perspectives on old age. The following excerpt is from* A Very Easy Death, *a profoundly moving, day-by-day account of the death of the author's mother. This deeply personal story reveals a face of de Beauvoir hitherto unknown.*

Sometimes, though very rarely, it happens that love, friendship or comradely feeling overcomes the loneliness of death: in spite of appearances, even when I was holding Maman's hand, I was not with her—I was lying to her. Because she had always been deceived, gulled, I found this ultimate deception revolting. I was making myself an accomplice of that fate which was so misusing her. Yet at the same time in every cell of my body I joined in her refusal, in her rebellion: and it was also because of that that her defeat overwhelmed me. Although I was not with Maman when she died, and although I had been with three people when they were actually dying, it was when I was at her bedside that I saw Death, the Death of the dance of death, with its bantering grin, the Death of fireside tales that knocks on the door, a scythe in its hand, the Death that comes from elsewhere, strange and inhuman: it had the very face of Maman when she showed her gums in a wide smile of unknowingness.

"He is certainly of an age to die." The sadness of the old; their banishment: most of them do not think that this age has yet come for them. I too made use of this cliché, and that when I was referring to my mother. I did not understand that one might sincerely weep for a relative, a grandfather aged seventy and more. If I met a woman of fifty overcome with sadness because she had just lost her mother, I thought her neurotic: we are all mortal; at eighty you are quite old enough to be one of the dead. . . .

But it is not true. You do not die from being born, nor from having lived, nor from old age. You die from *something*. The knowledge that because of her age my mother's life must soon come to an end did not lessen the horrible surprise: she had sarcoma. Cancer, thrombosis, pneumonia: it is as violent and unforeseen as an engine stopping in the middle of the sky. My mother encouraged one to be optimistic when, crippled with arthritis and dying, she asserted the infinite value of each instant; but her vain tenaciousness also ripped and tore the reassuring curtain of everyday triviality. There is no such thing as a natural death: nothing that happens to a man is ever natural, since his presence calls the world into question. All men must die: but for every man his death is an accident and, even if he knows it and consents to it, an unjustifiable violation. (pp. 37–38)

A DAUGHTER'S STORY

ROSE BIRD is the former Chief Justice of California. This article is adapted from an address to the nurses at Stanford University Hospital in honor of Nurses' Week, May 9, 1991.

Last April, Mother Nature outdid herself. Easter had just passed, and the sun enveloped the earth in its warmth. The flowers of spring were particularly breathtaking. And my mother was dying.

It began suddenly. My mother was having difficulty breathing, and her temperature was rising. The doctor decided to move her to Stanford Hospital. As they wheeled Mother to the ambulance, I raced to my car and followed.

I dreaded this hospital. Frankly, I associated it with my own vulnerability. Some fifteen years ago, I had my cancerous right breast removed at Stanford. At that time, I had had to come to terms with the possibility of my own death. And so I walked into the emergency room on that spring afternoon very much aware of the fragility of life.

For the first time, I faced the terrible possibility that Mother would never walk out of that building. Children, even middle-aged children, somehow never think their parents will die. However well you might prepare intellectually for the death of an elderly parent, you are never emotionally ready. I certainly was not.

I sat in the waiting room of the emergency area for what seemed like an eternity. A nurse approached and reassured me that I could see my mother in a few minutes. The nurse was pleasant and comforting at a moment that was anything but.

The doctors were trying to bring my mother's fibrillating heart into rhythm and stabilize her labile blood pressure. Several people were clustered around her gurney when I was finally allowed to see her. I was moved by their concern, and their patience with my questions. They let me speak to Mother to reassure her that I was close by. The doctor had elderly parents, and he was very gentle in introducing me to what was to come.

Finally, Mother was moved to the coronary care unit. When I saw her, she lay very still, her breathing still labored. The nurse, a tall redhead with a ready smile, looked like a commanding general in front of a battery of machines. She welcomed me and, as she worked, she began to explain what was happening and why. At that point, I knew mother was in capable hands, and for the first time that day I breathed more easily.

During the next eight days, I met many different nurses, with just as many personalities. There were some constants, however. Without exception, the nurses worked diligently and cheerfully. They explained what they were doing and why. And they were always honest about Mother's condition. I appreciated the fact that nothing was sugar-coated. Some nurses even took their break time to explain to me why certain decisions had to be made . . . why one course would be followed rather than another. While nursing Mother, they explained procedures and the meanings of the numbers the machines spewed out. They even let me help once in a while so I could feel useful.

A Role to Play. I felt I had a role in the process, and that is something for which I will be eternally grateful to the doctors and nurses who treated my mother. I never felt shut out, or that my questions were resented, or that alternatives were not explored.

When a patient's relatives are allowed to play some part in the treatment process, they feel less helpless. It is the life of a loved one that is at stake, and it is important to know that everything that could be done has been done for them . . . that the quality of their lives, as well as the quantity, has been weighed and considered. Patients and relatives need to feel that they have helped to make the decisions along with the medical team; that they are not pawns to be moved about at will, objects to be acted upon and manipulated. In my case, the doctors and nurses made me feel I was part of a team, that I had some responsibility, along with the professionals, for my mother's care and for the respect given her rights and her dignity.

One thing I never expected was the support system they set up to help me get through one of the most difficult times of my life.

Where did these wonderful people come from, so courteous and patient? They worked twelve-hour shifts on their feet, constantly monitoring the machines and taking care of Mother. And I thought of the news stories I had read about the low pay and long hours of nurses. Now that I could personally see what a stressful and demanding job they performed, both physically and mentally, I was embarrassed that I had taken so little time to understand their world.

Nurses know, I'm sure, that they have chosen a profession that demands industry, integrity, and compassion. The nurses whom I encountered also had a feeling for their craft . . . they cared enough about what they did to do it as well as they possibly could. They had a commitment to quality. It was clear that nursing, to them, was more than a job. It was a calling. People perform jobs to make money; nurses who care about their craft make a difference in the quality of people's lives.

I was struck by the ability of the nurses in the coronary care unit to keep their humanity in the middle of all the stress and strain. In many professions, the burden of work pressures can distort people's perception of the world and their development as human beings. For when others treat you as an object, there is a strong temptation to make them objects in return. And the competitive aspects of our society only reinforce the tendency to view life as a form of combat in which feelings are banished from the war zone and only the heartless survive. The nurses I knew resisted these temptations, this distortion—they were sensitive and caring human beings as well as skilled professionals.

By placing people in an environment that is supportive and caring, nurses help build a safety net so that people who are caught up in dealing with issues of life and death will not only learn about life, but will see the beauty that flows from a loving and caring community.

A Walk with Love and Death. During most of our lives, we deny, defy, or attempt to ignore the fact of death. We worship at the fountain of youth. We fool ourselves by creating the illusion that life is a permanent condition. And when we walk through a hospital's doors, almost all of us are ill equipped to handle what lies ahead. It's the doctors, and especially the nurses, who must help us face the fact that none of us is immortal.

For my mother, it was only a matter of time. With renal failure, pneumonia, haemophilus influenza, and heart complications, there was little hope. It was almost as if her body just gave up. Suddenly, I felt an overwhelming sadness, combined with a sense of helplessness. It was the nurse who helped me face the fact that, for the first time in my life, I had to seriously consider the possibility—yes, even the probability—that my mother, after 86 years, had only hours or days of life remaining.

Mother clung to life for another sixteen hours. I had promised her that she would not die alone and that I would stay with her as long as I was allowed to. I was sitting next to her bed when the numbers on the oxygenation machine began to decline—and then, quite suddenly, a big zero appeared on the screen. At first, I thought the position of the electrical patch was causing a malfunction. But the nurse's face and her outstretched hand spoke volumes. The doctor pronounced her dead at 4:20 A.M. on the morning of April 10.

The nurse embraced me and for a moment shared my overwhelming sorrow. Then she had to turn back to perform her final duty for my mother, one that I was allowed, again, to share. Together, the nurse and I bathed my mother's body.

With my farewells finally said, the nurse comforted me one last time. I picked up my purse and slowly walked out of the hospital into the chilly morning air. For the first time, I walked out into a world in which my mother no longer lived. My sense of loss was profound, and tears began to flow as I passed the beautiful tulip garden at the hospital's entrance.

As I walked, I thought how much my mother had taught me about life, about compassion and caring. And how in her death she had made it possible for me to see a community of skilled professionals who demonstrated in their everyday work the very best of what it means to be human and alive.

Here, in this small corner of Stanford, I had experienced what it was like to be in an environment where people mattered, where professionals were caring and compassionate, where I saw the very best of human nature. And, I thought, what greater gift could a loving mother give her child at the end of her life. (pp. 12–13)

LAMENT

EDNA ST. VINCENT MILLAY

Listen, children:
Your father is dead.
From his old coats
I'll make you little jackets;
I'll make you little trousers
From his old pants.
There'll be in his pockets
Things he used to put there,
Keys and pennies
Covered with tobacco;
Dan shall have the pennies
To save in his bank;
Anne shall have the keys
To make a pretty noise with.
Life must go on,
And the dead be forgotten;
Life must go on,
Though good men die;
Anne, Eat your breakfast;
Dan, take your medicine;
Life must go on;
I forget just why. (pp. 103–104)

The dying, too, have their roles to play and their duties to perform. Linfield, Hall, and Buchanan have gone to great pains to explain in the following selections.

How Do I Tell My Daughter?

Deborah Linfield was an attorney for the New York Times *who died June 3, 1992. She wrote this essay in November 1991.*

The Cleopatra's costume is barely put away. The candy isn't even half gone. And yet the annual ritual of choosing next year's costume has already begun. With all of the intenseness of an 8-year-old, she ponders, half to herself but half to me: Madonna? It's been done. A fairy princess? Too babyish. Pocahontas? Not politically correct. Usually, I listen to these ramblings with bemused enjoyment (after all, 8 is an awfully endearing age, as was 7 and 6 . . .). But this year everything is infused with a strange texture, a poignant overlay. I am her mother. Next year I may be dead.

A year ago I was diagnosed with inoperable cancer. I—who never so much as puffed on a cigarette—found myself with two thirty-something lungs riddled with disease. I've undergone every suggested form of chemotherapy (all more or less disgusting), but the disease is stubborn and refuses to disappear. Radiation and surgery are not options. Right now we're at a standoff, my tumors and I. But I know that won't last. Any day I expect my doctors to tell me that nothing else can be done, that it is only a matter of time.

This is everyone's nightmare. For me, the most horrible part of this disease is that it will take me from my daughter years too soon. I find myself accepting the likelihood of never seeing 40, but I cannot accept the thought of leaving her at this age.

I know children survive this sort of thing, and she's in an especially good position to (if there is such a thing). She is a happy, secure, self-possessed girl, popular with children and adults. She has a father and a soon-to-be stepfather who love her as much as I do and are an integral part of her life.

But she does not look to them in the same way. Mine is the hand she seeks to hold on a stroll. Mine is the office she calls first thing each day after school to relate her highs and lows. Mine is the opinion she seems to value most. Mine is the lap she climbs onto for comfort or a serious talk. The truth is, all feminist notions of equal parenting aside, that I am the anchor in her life. I am frantic that I won't be able to help her when my death tears her world apart.

Her alertness and sensitivity told her early on that something was wrong. And I have kept little from her. She's watched my hair fall out and my energy disappear. She's protested each trip to the hospital and greeted me with relief and joy on my return. She knows the medicine has not really worked and that I have to keep taking it even though it makes me sick. But it is obvious to me from the confident and joyous way she sallies forth each day that she has no thought that I will die soon.

What of our plans? She wants me to take her to Paris and the Greek isles and back to Disney World. She's counting the days until I let her pierce her ears—we've compromised on age 12. I made her a silent promise, one day when she was still in diapers, that I would help her with birth control when *she* needed it, not when her father or I thought she was of proper age. She's looking forward to starting junior high school, at my old school, and wants me to show her my old locker.

How will I ever explain it to her? How will I ever utter the words that Mommy has to die? She's never known more than transient unhappiness or pain. How will she deal with this—and why should she have to? How will we ever say goodbye?

When she was little and afraid of the dark, I would sit with her while she struggled to get to sleep. If I tried to tiptoe from her room too soon, she would call out reproachfully: "No go, Mama. No leave." And I would return to her bed, soothing her with the promise that I wasn't going anywhere. Occasionally still, sleep eludes her and she reverts to her babyish refrain. "Don't worry, sweetheart, I won't leave" is a lot harder to say these days, even though she and I are talking about different things.

Everything else about dying can be organized and rationalized. But this is so overwhelmingly tragic, so unremittingly painful, that my mind shuts down when I think of it. At times I think that the impossibility of saying goodbye—in and of itself—will cause this dreadful disease to give up and go bother someone else.

But of course I know that won't happen. And so we go on, sharing homework and dreams and bedtime stories and hugs, just as we always have—well, maybe with a bit more intensity on my part. Each evening as she dazzles me with her goodnight smile and drifts off to a peaceful sleep, I pray for a few more days before I have to tell her goodbye.

GAIL

STEPHEN S. HALL is a contributing editor to Health *and author of* Mapping the Next Millennium: The Discovery of New Geographies *(1992).*

Like most family tragedies, it came to life in one awful moment, and Ronald Watson, Sr., remembers it well. In the fall of 1986, Gail Farrow, his common-law wife, mother of their two boys and pregnant with their twins, came home from the prenatal clinic of Brigham and Women's Hospital in Boston. She came in the door with tears in her eyes, asked him to come into the bedroom. The hospital had tested her for AIDS, she said, and the test had come back positive.

For someone who had worked very hard to avoid slipping into the statistical ruts of the underclass, it was sourly ironic that Gail Farrow was destined to become one of the 81,000 Americans so far to perish of AIDS. Gail had grown up in a world where the role models were mostly roles to avoid. When she was about nine years old, she happened upon a woman in a hall of the Boston housing project where her family lived. This neighbor, as Gail later put it, "had many, many children by many different men." Gail watched as the woman shot up, saw the needle go into the woman's vein. That terrifying image never left her. She resolved that she would not succumb to drugs, that she would find a person she loved, that she would have one father for all her children. Modest goals, perhaps, but not for someone who left home for good at age 15 and ran the streets of Columbia Point and Roxbury, two of Boston's more notorious neighborhoods.

She was a strikingly lovely woman, with high cheekbones, proud eyes, and a fierce sense of self. She was also hard to read, stoic, not very trusting at first; but she was strong, and everybody gravitated toward that strength. She did things "gracefully and forcefully," a friend recalls, and that is exactly how she set out to create what she referred to as "a different life."

It began with Ronald Watson. Handsome and lithe, a smooth-skinned charmer with a wry, gentle smile on his face and an ever-present cap on his head, Ronald was not what you would call a role model in those days. He'd messed with drugs and drinking, had developed that same streetwise carapace necessary to survive. "If you ever let anyone know how much you hurt inside," he says now, much mellowed by fatherhood and mourning, "they would take advantage of it."

Gail and Ronald let down their respective guards long enough to fall in love. In the summer of 1981, Ronald got a job driving an ice cream truck. He would pick up Gail at the drug counseling clinic where she worked and they would sell ice cream around Columbia Point. The business became a courtship; the courtship led to a family.

In 1982, Gail gave birth to Ronald, Jr., and a year later came Frank. In 1983 too came a bout with cancer, which required hospitalization, surgery, blood transfusions, and a lengthy, painful convalescence. But by 1986 Gail was working again, and was pregnant with the twins. The family had moved into Roxbury's Mission Hill project. Drug dealers openly hawked crack on the street, and Gail's children, perched in their second-floor window, gazed down on hopheads and petty thieves. No matter. Gail chased the pushers away, declaring theirs the only "drug-free doorway" in the project.

And then it all came crashing down: a recurrence of cancer, the AIDS test, a prognosis you could learn from a newspaper headline. (Gail apparently became infected from the transfusions in 1983). She who hated to trust others now found herself at the mercy of the health care system.

"There wasn't a real bond at first," says James Maguire, her physician at Brigham and Women's Hospital. "She came across as a streetwise product of a pretty tough part of Boston. She had her own grammar, which was not the best, so the initial, misleading impression was of someone with not a lot of education and not too smart. And the truth was, she was sharp as nails. You couldn't slip anything by her."

Gail refused to deal with insensitive doctors, refused rooms on hospital floors if she didn't like the nurses, knew more about her disease than some of the interns. She was "non-compliant," in the jargon of the doctors—she checked herself out of the hospital against medical advice to be with her family, even on as little a pretext as having to buy milk for her children. But Maguire deferred to her judgment and her determination. "If I went up against her," Maguire says, "I knew I wouldn't win."

Only slowly did it dawn on her doctor, her nurses, her devoted and growing support group, that the family kept Gail alive. Dragging her intravenous pole from room to room, she cooked and cleaned, washed and ironed, planned the birthday parties, organized trips to the fair. "I don't have time to think about dying," she would say. "I have to think of my family." She complained rarely, despite the pneumonias and blood transfusions, the 17 hospitalizations and dozens of emergency room visits. "Why me?" she once confided to Claire Welch, the social worker who befriended her at the hospital. "I would be the one to put pumpkins in the window at Halloween, when other mothers didn't even know it was Halloween, they were so high."

By the summer of 1989, Gail weighed barely 100 pounds. She couldn't swallow food. Day after day she was confined to bed with the chills she called "the riders."

Toward the end there were many things on her mind. Deciding whether she had the strength to visit her sister-in-law Vanessa, who lay dying of kidney and liver failure in a hospital in Framingham. Ordering a plaque to honor James Maguire. Lowering the boom on Ronald one final time, for he had drifted back to heroin during her illness (checked every six months, he has repeatedly tested negative for the AIDS virus).

She prepared beautiful, loving letters to her husband and sons. She made a videotape at the hospital. She discussed her funeral service with the priest, insisting that the nature of her illness be described, its prevention specifically discussed. And at the end of October, lying in the back seat of Ronald's rundown Buick during the ride out to Framingham, she managed to visit Ronald's sister Vanessa. "They was real close," he says, "and they told us that they were going to die the same day."

That is why, when the phone rang around 9:30 on the morning of November 10, 1989, and Ronald picked it up and listened to the voice telling him that his sister had died, his thoughts went instantly, fearfully, to Gail. She lay in bed at home in a coma, barely hanging on. After consulting with doctors, Ronald and the home-care nurse disconnected her intravenous line. Relatives gathered a final time.

"She was fading deeper and deeper," Ronald recalls. "I got into bed with her and made her some promises. I promised to get the plaque for Doctor Maguire. I promised to take care of the kids. And I promised to stay straight. Doc Maguire said her hearing would be the last thing to go, and I told her I loved her. I felt her hand squeeze mine." The last to come home that afternoon were the boys. "She seemed to wait until her kids, her mother, and her sisters were there. After her sons came, then she left. She died with a smile." He holds the memory like a worry stone, testing its firmness, satisfied with its substance. "She died with a *big* smile."

Gail Farrow died that November afternoon, but as was her habit, she'd done her Christmas shopping in July. Everybody who had helped her—doctor, home-care nurses, social worker, nutritionist—received presents. James Maguire received a shirt, a sweater, and the plaque of appreciation. He also discovered a new way of thinking about patients. "I learned to let the patient have a *much* more active role in decisions. Not in technical things like drug treatment, but where the treatment takes place, the length of hospitalization, whether certain procedures should be performed. I learned that you can really do a lot more outside the hospital than I ever thought was possible."

Claire Welch, the social worker, received figurines of two children ("To remind you of my sons," Gail wrote) and the understanding that "non-compliance" in patients could be a form of emotional health. "The other thing I learned from Gail is to hang in there. If I had picked up on her earliest vibes, I might not have gotten so involved."

Ronald received that last smile. "She was holding on because she knew I could do it, but she just wasn't sure. The smile on her face told me that everything I done was okay. Gail being the person she was is what made me able to do it."

Months after Gail's death, Ronald Watson slouches in a living-room chair, staring through the stubborn haze of mourning. On the wall behind him are school certificates: perfect attendance for Frank and Ronald, Jr., good sportsmanship and effort for Ronald, Jr. Three-year-old Benny drags a white blanket in from the bedroom. His twin, Kenny, knocks over a plastic dish of cheese snacks. (Although Gail had AIDS while pregnant with the twins, they are not infected.) The family sometimes seems as precarious as that tottering plastic bowl, but Ronald has, according to the social workers helping him, risen to the challenge magnificently.

When there is a moment of respite, Ronald inserts the video tape into the VCR, freezes the frame on Gail's face, and then reads the words she left behind: "I can die knowing you are in charge and that gives me peace. I hope you and our sons will be close and support each other. You will get a lot from them, too. I wish I could be there to see how beautiful they are when they grow up. Let them use you as a role model. . . ." (pp. 62–69)

The Face of a Wolf

James H. Buchanan

This whole business of dying is so completely misunderstood by the living. The assorted visitors, well-wishers, bereaved family members, curious doctors, distracted nurses, angry attendants that one receives throughout the day are but travelers in a foreign country. They enter the court and kingdom of the patient but only on official business of import and export; they tarry not nor do they adopt the local customs of the country within which they find themselves. Indeed, there is an arrogance, even an insolence to these tourists which is the insulation by which they protect themselves against the contamination of death. After all, what do they know of pain, sweat, incontinence, putrefaction of rotting flesh, and the sheer humiliation of not being able to control your bladder and bowels? They measure your fever, but they do not suffer it. They study your blood, but they do not bleed it. They palpate your liver, your spleen, your guts; but they do not feel them. They hear your heart and yet cannot feel its weakened beat; they measure your blood pressure and yet cannot feel its intensity; they peer, with curious abandon, into the various interstices, holes, canyons, craters of your body and yet are never part of the great cavern you have become. They are guests, not residents of this house of death which you inhabit. How then could they possibly understand?

In the evenings, they go home to husbands, wives, friends, or lovers. Cool and comfortable in their freedom from pain and disease, they lounge in languid, lazy luxury and finally curl up in front of the television or in one another's arms. And later, in their beds and surrounded by darkness, they drink freely and deeply from one another's flesh. Their strong, muscled loins arch and twist with intense pleasures far beyond your own diminished recall while yours instead quiver with an agony born of death rather than orgasms issuing from life. Later, lying in one another's arms, they are renewed while you are depleted; they sleep well and soundly while you dream dreams of death and frightful, hideous sights. In the morning they enter once again into the ever diminishing circumference of your dying light.

They ask you how you slept without waiting for the answer. They hope that you are feeling better today although they know that you are not. It is small talk, simply chatter intended to break the boredom and monotony of their required and enforced visit. You, in turn, are polite, casual, and self-effacing. They already know of your pain, of your dying, of your fear, and of your agony. And so why mention it? They know already that you are worse today than you were yesterday and worse yesterday than the day before. And so why mention it? When asked how you are feeling, why not simply agree that you are fine? Does it matter; could it make a difference? It is a game, an elaborate series of gestures and half-truths intended to make the visitor feel comfortable in the presence of death. After all, it is the privilege and the obligation of the dying not to alarm or unduly frighten the living. Thus, the entrance of every visitor for whatever reason must be handled delicately and precisely. After all, you are dying and they are busy. Be careful not to disarm them with stark realities, truths too cruel for the light of day, or hysterical scenes of fear and remorse. They have come into your room, specifically to your room and to no other, to be entertained! Do not forsake your obligations as host and guestmaster.

The living will inquire of the dying about their conditions of living. "Are you comfortable; do you have enough to eat and is it good?" Perhaps they will even make a little joke about the hospital food. Laugh along with them and agree that it is not so very good. They will, of course, tell you that you look good—much too good to be sick—and that they wished they looked half as well. Do not become angry; it is an innocent little game and you should, out of respect and obligation, play along with them. Soon now they will depart, for the atmosphere is becoming oppressive and they have discharged their obligations, and you should thank them very much for coming, confess that you actually feel better after their visit, and invite them back again. Out in the hallway you will hear their rushed and whispering voices disappearing down the corridor, and you cannot avoid the fragmentations of meaning that float like nuclear fallout back to your room. "Dying . . . God, she looks so bad . . . only a few days left they say . . . did you see her eyes? . . . Myra says that she is . . ." (pp. 141–143)

DEATH

JOHN STONE's work includes In All This Rain, *a poetry collection, from which this excerpt comes.*

I have seen come on
slowly as rust
sand

or suddenly as when
someone leaving
a room

finds the doorknob
come loose in his hand

A GENEROUS DEATH

*ELLEN D. BAER is an associate professor at the University of Penn-
sylvania School of Nursing. A recent article, "The Feminist Disdain for Nursing," recently appeared in the* New York Times *and
is excerpted below.*

The day before he died, the last time I saw him, my brother blew
me a kiss as I left his hospital room. At first I didn't know what
he was doing—lifting his hand so haltingly, moving it, wavering,
towards his face. I thought he was calling me back, maybe wanting something. He couldn't speak. The kaposi tumors on the roof
of his mouth prevented enunciation and increased salivation to
the point that he had ceased trying to talk. His gestures had become all-important and this one stopped me in the doorway,
catching me as I glanced back. Then his hand brushed his lips
and stretched towards me and I realized it was a kiss—a wonderful, loving, generous kiss that stays near my heart always,
ready to remember and treasure. It meant so much to me—a
farewell salute, sibling forgiveness, recognition of efforts made,
and a promise of future hope—from my baby brother, childhood pal, and Irish twin, dying from AIDS at age 48.

ONLY HUMAN

*LU CARTER, a nurse from Norfolk, Nebraska, wrote this poem
that appeared in the July 1991 issue of* The Western Journal of
Medicine.

i was glad
i had taken the time
to hold the dead man's head in my hands
and comb his hair
even though i am always afraid
combing the dead fibers
will make them fall out

and i was glad
i had rolled a towel
and placed it under his gaping jaw

and that i had arranged the crisp white sheet
smoothly and neatly
across his motionless chest

for when she asked through tear-filled eyes
if she could see him and say good-bye
all i could do was nod my head
and hope my eyes were communicating the words
wedged so snugly in my throat

A nurse who has made a career of working with the dying has synopsized her experiences with profound simplicity in this final selection on dying and grieving.

LISTENING TO THE DYING

JOY K. UFEMA, Pennsylvania nurse and pioneer in the nursing care of dying patients, credits an Elisabeth Kübler-Ross seminar with giving her career this focus. She has appeared on "60 Minutes" and has written a book about her experiences working with the dying: Brief Companions. *The following excerpt is from her biography in Schorr and Zimmerman's* Making Choices, Taking Chances.

Abraham Maslow said the self-actualized person simply finds out what he does right and does it.

My affinity to dying patients led me to read and study. I signed up to go to a seminar conducted by Elisabeth Kübler-Ross.

Sitting among 2,000 participants, I suddenly saw myself standing at a podium, lecturing to hundreds of people about *my* experiences of working with dying patients and their families.

This imagery and self-fulfilling prophecy would soon serve me quite successfully.

I attended workshops and seminars, read lots of books, studied theories, and then sorted out for myself what I felt was good and valuable.

I spent more time with terminally ill patients—listening. I visited before and after my regular shift. Within a few weeks, I realized this work was tenfold more rewarding for me than regular nursing.

Never having been the kind of person to sit back and wait for opportunity to knock, I decided to *make* something happen. I approached . . . the director of nursing, and asked if I could have a job working exclusively with the dying patients throughout the hospital.

She said yes. She had also heard the challenge of Kübler-Ross, and, after all, not many young nurses were bombarding her with this request.

One of the most difficult adjustments for me was to learn to sit down and stop "fussing" over the patients.

I recall the first morning that I worked as a "nurse-specialist in death and dying." I had worked ten days in a row on the urology floor and had five more days to put in before my first weekend off in a long time. Yet, I had energy to spare!

My patient was a 19-year-old with cancer of the testicle. It had metastasized to his lung. His night nurse had given him a bath and changed his linens. He was resting.

At 8 AM I introduced myself.

"Tom, my name is Joy, and I'm working with the patients here who are seriously ill. Do you feel like talking about anything?"

"Not right this minute, but you could hang around if you don't have anybody else who needs you right now."

After 20 minutes of "hanging around" his bedside, I felt terribly uncomfortable—not with death, but with my need to do something. I had fluffed his pillow, examined his IV site, gotten fresh juice, and done several other busy things.

Wearily, Tom took my hand and said, "Look, Joy, I don't really need any nurse stuff right now, but it sure would feel good just to have you sit here beside me."

I got his message.

I sat.

He dozed.

The nurses stared.

I felt comfortable.

I learned a profound lesson from Tom: dying persons know exactly what is best for themselves. If they don't come right out and tell you, you have to ask.

"What do you want?"

"What can I do that will help?"

The days turned into years—good, hard-working years. (pp. 360–361)

X

ON MAKING A DIFFERENCE

*𝒴*ou see things; and you say, "Why?" But I dream
things that never were; and I say, "Why not?"

George Bernard Shaw, *Back to Methuselah,* 1921

A popular volume edited by Thelma Schorr and Anne Zimmerman and containing autobiographical sketches of contemporary nurse leaders is called *Making Choices, Taking Chances* (1988),
a title encapsulating the themes of the lives portrayed. After reading this chapter of writing by and about people who made a difference within various spheres of influence, one might reaffirm
that such a title says it all. But a third critical dimension stands
out in the literature presented here—having vision, having a
dream. Thus, the strong pieces in this collection are about having
vision, making choices, taking chances and changing the world—
through personal, clinical, or political acts, in small corners or in
all corners, for a moment or for generations to come. As we might
expect, the chapter opens with motivational literature, with writing or public speaking that, through the force of its expression or

message, moves people to think, to hope, to act; and it closes with testimonials to their effect.

* * *

The attitudes with which "difference-makers" approach the world and their daily lives are inspiring to those touched by their words.

FOR THOSE WHO NURSE

For us who Nurse, our Nursing is a thing, which, unless we are making progress every year, every month, every week . . . we are going back.

Florence Nightingale, 1872

OUT OF MY LIFE AND THOUGHT

ALBERT SCHWEITZER (1875–1965), French philosopher, physician, musician, author, founded a missionary hospital in Lambarene (present-day Gabon) where he spent much of his life. In 1953 he was awarded the Nobel Peace Prize. The following passage is taken from the Epilogue to Out of My Life and Thought, *1931.*

To the question whether I am a pessimist or an optimist, I answer that my knowledge is pessimistic, but my willing and hoping are optimistic.

I am pessimistic in that I experience in its full weight what we conceive to be the absence of purpose in the course of world happenings. Only at quite rare moments have I felt really glad to be alive. I could not but feel with a sympathy full of regret all the pain that I saw around me, not only that of men but that of the whole creation. From this community of suffering I have never tried to withdraw myself. It seemed to me a matter of course that we should all take our share of the burden of pain which lies upon the world. Even while I was a boy at school it was clear to me that no explanation of the evil in the world could ever satisfy me; all explanations, I felt, ended in sophistries, and at bottom had no other object than to make it possible for men to share in the misery around them, with less keen feelings. . . .

But however much concerned I was at the problem of the misery in the world, I never let myself get lost in broodings over it; I always held firmly to the thought that each one of us can do a little to bring some portion of it to an end. Thus I came gradually to rest content in the knowledge that there is only one thing we can understand about the problem, and that is that each of us has to go his own way, but as one who means to help to bring about deliverance.

In my judgment, too, of the situation in which mankind finds itself at the present time I am pessimistic. I cannot make myself believe that that situation is not so bad as it seems to be, but I am inwardly conscious that we are on a road which, if we continue to tread it, will bring us into "Middle Ages" of a new character. The spiritual and material misery to which mankind of today is delivering itself through its renunciation of thinking and of the ideals which spring therefrom, I picture to myself in its utmost compass. And yet I remain optimistic. One belief of my childhood I have preserved with the certainty that I can never lose it: belief in truth. I am confident that the spirit generated by truth is stronger than the force of circumstances. In my view no other destiny awaits mankind than that which, through its mental and spiritual disposition, it prepares for itself. Therefore I do not believe that it will have to tread the road to ruin right to the end.

If men can be found who revolt against the spirit of thoughtlessness, and who are personalities sound enough and profound enough to let the ideals of ethical progress radiate from them as a force, there will start an activity of the spirit which will be strong enough to evoke a new mental and spiritual disposition in mankind.

Because I have confidence in the power of truth and of the spirit, I believe in the future of mankind. Ethical acceptance of the world contains within itself an optimistic willing and hoping which can never be lost. It is, therefore, never afraid to face the dismal reality, and to see it as it really is. (pp. 240–241)

THREE GUINEAS

VIRGINIA WOOLF (1882–1941) was an English author whose work includes novels such as Mrs. Dalloway, To the Lighthouse, *short stories, and essay collections such as* A Room of One's Own.

We are here, on the bridge, to ask ourselves certain questions. And they are very important questions; and we have very little time in which to answer them. The questions that we have to ask and to answer about the procession during this moment of transition are so important that they may well change the lives of all men and women forever. For we have to ask ourselves, here and now, do we wish to join that procession, or don't we? On what terms shall we join that process? Above all, where is it leading us, the procession of educated men? The moment is short; it may last five years; ten years, or perhaps only a matter of a few months longer. But the questions must be answered; and they are so important that if all the daughters of educated men did nothing, from morning to night, but consider that procession, from every angle, if they did nothing but ponder it and analyze it, and think about it and read about it and pool their thinking and reading, and what they see and what they guess, their time would be better spent than in any other activity now open to them.

. . . Let us never cease from thinking—what is this "civilization" in which we find ourselves? What are these ceremonies and why should we take part in them? What are these professions and why should we make money out of them? Where in short is it leading us, the procession of the sons of educated men? (pp. 62–63)

HABITS OF THE HEART

R. BELLAH ET AL. A community volunteer, who was a research subject in the 1985 study, Habits of the Heart, *is quoted in part in the following excerpt.*

One does not . . . give simply in order to get. One's reward for such giving is not simply a good feeling, not simply the company of like-minded friends. It is an experience that enfolds and somehow makes meaningful a tremendous amount of pain, frustration, and indeed loneliness. "Of course I feel lonely. I would be lying if I said I didn't. People who are willing to love are always going to be lonely—that's what you are going to have to cope with. I'm lonely all the time. It goes with the territory. My husband feels lonely. We've supported one another even when that means sharing our lonely feelings. We are a very close, supportive family, private about certain things. But this ability to support one another is something that I, my husband, my kids, and only a few other people I know have—a generosity of spirit in which you are willing to invest emotional commitment in other people and other things. A lot of people can't live that way. That doesn't mean that I don't respect them or love them less for it. You will find this spirit in most people involved in community work—and in some politicians.

Generosity of spirit is thus the ability to acknowledge an interconnectedness—one's "debts to society"—that binds one to others whether one wants to accept it or not. It is also the ability to engage in the caring that nurtures that interconnectedness. It is a virtue that everyone should strive for, even though few people have a lot of it—a virtue the practice of which gives meaning to the frustration of political work and the inevitable loneliness of the separate self. It is a virtue that leads one into community work and politics and is sustained by such involvements. (p. 194)

Many of those who have written profound passages about the search for meaning in life and the means of making a difference are women. Read below the words of women of many cultures.

IN SEARCH OF THE SELF AS HERO

NELLIE WONG, born in Oakland, California's Chinatown, is a feminist poet and writer. She is active in The Freedom Socialist Party and Radical Women. Her work has appeared in many journals and anthologies including The Forbidden Stitch *in 1989 and*

This Bridge Called My Back *(1983), from which this passage is taken.*

You believed once in your own passivity, your own powerlessness, your own spiritual malaise. You are now awakening in the beginnings of a new birth. Not born again, but born for the first time, triumphant and resolute, out of experience and struggle, out of a flowing, living memory, out of consciousness and will, facing, confronting, challenging head-on the contradictions of your lives and the lives of people around you. You believe now in the necessity and beauty of struggle: that feminism for you means working for the equality and humanity of women and men, for children, for the love that is possible.

You rub your legs in this cold room. You shiver when you recall your own self-pity when you had no date on New Year's Eve, when you regretted the family gathering because it reminded you that you stood out, a woman without a man, a woman without children. Now you are strengthened, encouraged by the range of your own experiences as a writer, a feminist, an organizer, a secretary. Now you are fired by your own needs, by the needs of your sisters and brothers in the social world, by your journey toward solidarity, against tyranny in the workplace, on the streets, in our literature and in our homes.

You are fueled by the clarity of your own sight, heated by your own energy to assert yourselves as a human being, a writer, a woman, an Asian American, a feminist, a clerical worker, a student, a teacher, not in loneliness and isolation, but in a community of freedom fighters. Your poems and stories will do some of the work for you, but poems and stories alone aren't enough. Nothing for you is ever enough and so you challenge yourselves, again and again, to try something new, to help build a movement, to organize for the rights of working people, to write a novel, a play, to create a living theater that will embody your dreams and vision, energy in print, on stage, at work that will assert the will of an independent, freedom-loving woman, that will reflect a sensibility of Asian America, of feminism, of sharing food and wealth with all the people, with all your kin.

And you will not stop working and writing because you care, because you refuse to give up, because you won't submit to the forces that will silence you, a cheong hay poa, a long steam woman, a talker, a dancer who moves with lightning. And you are propelled by your sense of fair play, by your respect for the dead and the living, by your . . . American laughter and language, by your desire to help order the chaotic world that you live in, knowing as the stars sparkle on this New Year's night that you will not survive the work that still needs to be done in the streets of Gold Mountain. (pp. 180–181)

OUT OF THE HARD PLACES

CARRIE LENBURG has long been an advocate of nontraditional education, serving as the first director of New York's External Degree Nursing Program (now known as the Regents College Degrees Program). Her writing has appeared in books and academic journals. This poem is taken from her biography in Schorr and Zimmerman's Making Choices, Taking Chances.

Out of the hard places
I learn to be born again
for part of me dies inside
when I experience defeat and rejection.

Out of the hard places
I learn who I am,
where I have been
and where I yet can go. (p. 205)

WOMEN'S CONSCIOUSNESS, MAN'S WORLD

SHEILA ROWBOTHAM is a socialist writer whose work includes Women's Consciousness, Man's World *(1973), excerpted here.*

The oppressed without hope are mysteriously quiet. When the conception of change is beyond the limits of the possible, there are no words to articulate discontent so it is sometimes held not to exist. This mistaken belief arises because we can only hear silence in the moment in which it is breaking. (p. 29)

OF WOMAN BORN

ADRIENNE RICH *is excerpted here from her work* Of Woman Born: Motherhood as Experience and Institution, *1976.*

The most notable fact that culture imprints on women is the sense of our limits. The most important thing one woman can do for another is to illuminate and expand her sense of actual possibilities. For a mother this means more than contending with the reductive images of females in children's books, movies, television, the schoolroom. It means that the mother herself is trying to expand the limits of her life. *To refuse to be a victim:* and then go from there. (p. 246)

IF YOU CAN WALK

DORIS ARMSTRONG *is the President of the Council of Graduates of Foreign Nursing Schools.*

IF YOU CAN WALK . . . YOU CAN DANCE
IF YOU CAN TALK . . . YOU CAN SING

That is a saying from Zimbabwe. I first saw it printed above a drawing of two strong African women, clasping hands in dance. Under the picture, someone had written, NO EXCUSES!

IF YOU CAN WALK . . . YOU CAN DANCE

Nurses throughout the world could take these words as our credo. Certainly, as a profession, we have insisted on *seeing possibilities,* on *realizing potential.* We have done this as we cared for the ill and injured. We have done this as we moved into the world of administration, research, and education. We have done this as we ventured to speak in the halls of government on behalf of the young, the poor, the sick, the disenfranchised.

In our efforts to encourage our patients, our students, our legislators not to be satisfied with walking when dance is possible, we have shown the way. Like the women in the picture, nurses have demonstrated that the dance that embodies our vision of the future is not a solo performance. It is a group dance—strong individuals joining each other, the weight and force of individual momentum, balanced in the effort of the group.

WHAT TO DO FROM HERE AND HOW

GLORIA EVANGELINA ANZALDÚA calls herself a Chicana poet, una mestiza, and a teacher of the children of migrant workers. In 1981 she co-edited a groundbreaking anthology of feminist writings, This Bridge Called My Back: Writings by Radical Women of Color. *The passage below is from the Foreword to the 2nd edition of that book, subtitled* Kitchen Table *(1983).*

Perhaps like me you are tired of suffering and talking about suffering, estás hasta el pescuezo de sufrimiento, de contar las lluvias de sangre pero no las lluvias de flores (up to your neck with suffering, of counting the rains of blood but not the rains of flowers). Like me you may be tired of making a tragedy of our lives. A abandonar ese autocanibalismo: coraje, tristeza, miedo (let's abandon this autocannibalism: rage, sadness, fear). Basta de gritar contra el viento—toda palabra es ruido si no está acompañada de acción (enough of shouting against the wind—all words are noise if not accompanied with action). Dejemos hablar hasta que hagamos la palabra luminosa y activa (let's work not talk, let's say nothing until we've made the world luminous and active). Basta de pasividad y de pasatiempo mientras esperamos al novio, a la novio, a la Diosa, o a la Revolución (enough of passivity and passing time while waiting for the boy friend, the girl friend, the Goddess, or the Revolution). No nos podemos quedar paradas con los brazos cruzados en medio del puente (we can't afford to stop in the middle of the bridge with arms crossed).

And yet to act is not enough. Many of us are learning to sit perfectly still, to sense the presence of the Soul and commune with

Her. We are beginning to realize that we are not wholly at the mercy of circumstance, nor are our lives completely out of our hands. That if we posture as victims we will be victims, that hopelessness is suicide, that self-attacks stop us in our tracks. We are slowly moving past the resistance within, leaving behind the defeated images. We have come to realize that we are not alone in our struggles nor separate nor autonomous but that we—white black straight queer female male—are connected and interdependent. We are each accountable for what is happening down the street, south of the border or across the sea. And those of us who have more of anything: brains, physical strength, political power, spiritual energies, are learning to share them with those that don't have. We are learning to depend more and more on our own sources for survival, learning not to let the weight of this burden, the bridge, break our backs. Haven't we always borne jugs of water, children, poverty? Why not learn to bear baskets of hope, love, self-nourishment and to step lightly?

With This Bridge . . . hemos comenzado a salir de las sombras; hemos comenzado a reventar rutina y costumbres opresivas y a levantar los tabues; hemos comenzado a acarrear con orgullo la tarea de deshelar corazones y cambiar conciencias (we have begun to come out of the shadows; we have begun to break with routines and oppressive customs and to discard taboos; we have commenced to carry with pride the task of thawing hearts and changing consciousness). Mujeres, a no dejar que el peligro del viaje y de la inmensidad del territorio nos asuste—a mirar hacia adelante y abrir paso en el monte (Women, let's not let the danger of the journey and the vastness of the territory scare us—let's look forward and open paths in these woods). Caminante, no hay puentes, se hace puentes al andar (Voyager, there are no bridges, one builds them as one walks). (pp. iv–v)

WE ARE THE ONES

AURORA LEVINS MORALES is a Jewish-Puerto Rican writer whose works include a remarkable prose-poem on anti-Semitism, "If I Forget Thee, Oh Jerusalem," in Getting Home Alive *(1986).*

This excerpt is taken from her essay, ". . . And Even Fidel Can't Change That!" in This Bridge Called My Back; Kitchen Table *(1983).*

> If we're the ones who can imagine it,
> if we're the ones who dream about it,
> if we're the ones who need it most,
> then no one else can do it.

> We're the ones.

They Came to Stay

Maya Angelou rose from a childhood of poverty in Stamps, Arkansas, to become one of America's most heralded poets. In January 1993, she read her poem "On the Pulse of Morning" at the inauguration of President Clinton. I Know Why the Caged Bird Sings, *the first of several books, described her painful childhood and revealed a woman of extraordinary talents. She wrote the following passage in her introduction to* I Dream a World *(1989), a collection of photo essays honoring African American women whose ancestors were brought to the United States beginning in 1619.*

The heartbreaking tenderness of Black women *and* their majestic strength speak of the heroic survival of a people who were stolen into subjugation, denied chastity, and refused innocence.

These women have descended from grandmothers and great-grandmothers who knew the lash first-hand, and to whom protection was a phantom known of but seldom experienced. Their faces are captured here for the ages to regard and wonder, but they are whole women. Their hands have brought children through blood to life, nursed the sick, and folded the winding cloths. Their wombs have held the promise of a race which has proven in each challenging century that despite threat and mayhem it has come to stay. Their feet have trod the shifting swampland of insecurity, yet they have tried to step neatly onto the footprints of mothers who went before. They are not apparitions; they are not superwomen. Despite their majestic struggle they are not larger than life. Their humanness is evident in their accessibility.

ANNA ARNOLD HEDGEMAN

ANNA ARNOLD HEDGEMAN was the first woman to serve in the cabinet of a mayor of New York. Her role as a member of the cabinet of Mayor Robert Wagner from 1954 to 1958 was preceded and followed by work with governmental and civic organizations, both national and international. The following excerpt is also from I Dream a World.

I'm my father's daughter. I'm a product of 1865 as well as 1900. He had come out of the slave system. His mother and father had been slaves and they were in our household in Saint Paul, Minnesota. . . .

Eleanor Roosevelt was the first unelected woman president of these United States. When the war came, the Negro nurse had an awful time getting into the whole thing to take care of her men whom the others were not going to take care of. It was known that that was true. We were worried and I wanted to see Mrs. Roosevelt. I sat in the second row where she was speaking and then I made myself last in the receiving line. I had my sentence ready. "Mrs. Roosevelt, the Negro nurse is being cheated by our government in terms of the war effort, and I need to talk with you." She looked at me and said, "Of course," and invited the organizers for tea at her apartment. Believe it or not, within two weeks things began to happen. She knew people. (p. 90)

The following two selections are an interesting contrast, the first a bold challenge to nurses, the second a poetic parable about risk-taking.

THE NURSE AS A REVOLUTIONARY

JOSEPH A. CALIFANO, JR. served as Secretary of Health, Education and Welfare under President Jimmy Carter, initiating extensive reorganization of HEW and introducing major initiatives on immunization, smoking and alcoholism. He has authored eight books, the most recent of which is The Triumph and Tragedy of Lyndon Johnson: The White House Years.

What a time to be part of the American health care system! There is a revolution afoot as profound, in its way, as the revolution in the Soviet Union that is shaking the world. And American nurses have the chance to be American health care revolutionaries. . . .

The Nurse's Responsibility

Each of us is important in the effort [to reform health care]— doctors, hospital administrators, pharmaceutical companies, government legislators and administrators, medical equipment manufacturers, and patients. But few of us have a greater responsibility or opportunity than the American nurse. Revolutions, like nations, do not drift in a vacuum. They move in a direction. And in the coming years, the opportunity for nurses to help shape the direction of America's health care revolution is enormous.

In health care delivery and policy today, the Administration and the Congress, the states and the cities, employers and unions, providers and purchasers are floundering. They are thrashing about like children who find themselves for the first time in water over their heads, scared about where they are, not knowing in which direction to swim, certain only that they do not want to drown.

The issue for your profession is whether nurses will choose to sit on the sidelines or position themselves to help lead the revolution. . . . (pp. 14–15)

THE TWO GRETELS

ROBIN MORGAN, feminist poet and author, is editor of Ms *magazine; her books include* Sisterhood Is Global *and* Upstairs in the Garden, *a collection of poems.*

The two Gretels were exploring the forest.
Hansel was home,
sending up flares.

Sometimes one Gretel got afraid.
She said to the other Gretel,
"I think I'm afraid."
"Of course we are," Gretel replied.

Sometime the other Gretel whispered,
with a shiver,
"You think we should turn back?"
To which her sister Gretel answered,
"We can't. We forgot the breadcrumbs."

So, they went forward
because
they simply couldn't imagine the way back.

And eventually, they found the Gingerbread House,
and the Witch, who was really, they discovered,
The Great Good Mother Goddess,
and they all lived happily ever after

The Moral of this story is:
Those who would have the whole loaf,
let alone the House,
had better throw away their breadcrumbs.

It is the holders of the vision who, if powerfully spoken, create the tide of rising expectations that carries a people or a profession to new heights. Martin Luther King epitomized that tradition. Such literature resounds in the ears and heart of the reader and provokes a restlessness throughout the soul.

MARTIN LUTHER KING, JR. (1929–1968), American minister and charismatic leader of the civil rights movement, was committed to nonviolent tactics toward achieving integration and equality for all Americans. In 1964 he won the Nobel Peace Prize; in 1968, he was assassinated in Memphis, Tennessee.

Trumpet of Conscience

If we do not act, we shall surely be dragged down the long, dark and shameful corridor of time reserved for those who possess power without compassion, might without morality, and strength without sight.

> Dr. King delivered his now-immortal "I Have a Dream" speech at the great civil rights march that ended at the Lincoln Memorial, Washington, DC, August 28, 1963.

I Have a Dream

Five score years ago, a great American, in whose symbolic shadow we stand, signed the Emancipation Proclamation. This momentous decree came as a great beacon light of hope to millions of Negro slaves who had been seared in the flames of withering injustice. It came as a joyous daybreak to end the long night of captivity.

But one hundred years later, we must face the tragic fact that the Negro is still not free. One hundred years later, the life of the Negro is still sadly crippled by the manacles of segregation and the chains of discrimination. One hundred years later, the Negro lives on a lonely island of poverty in the midst of a vast ocean of material prosperity. One hundred years later, the Negro is still languishing in the corners of American society and finds himself an exile in his own land. So we have come here today to dramatize an appalling condition.

In a sense we have come to our nation's capital to cash a check. When the architects of our republic wrote the magnificent words of the Constitution and the Declaration of Independence, they were signing a promissory note to which every American was to fall heir. This note was a promise that all men would be guaranteed the unalienable rights of life, liberty, and the pursuit of happiness.

It is obvious today that America has defaulted on this promissory note insofar as her citizens of color are concerned. Instead of honoring this sacred obligation, America has given the Negro people a bad check; a check which has come back marked "insufficient funds." But we refuse to believe that the bank of justice is bankrupt. We refuse to believe that there are insufficient funds in the great vaults of opportunity of this nation. So we have come to cash this check—a check that will give us upon demand the riches of freedom and the security of justice.

We have also come to this hallowed spot to remind America of the fierce urgency of *now*. This is no time to engage in the luxury of cooling off or to take the tranquilizing drug of gradualism. *Now* is the time to make real the promises of democracy. *Now* is the time to rise from the dark and desolate valley of segregation to the sunlit path of racial justice. *Now* is the time to open the doors of opportunity to all of God's children. *Now* is the time to lift our nation from the quicksands of racial injustice to the solid rock of brotherhood.

It would be fatal for the nation to overlook the urgency of the moment and to underestimate the determination of the Negro. This sweltering summer of the Negro's legitimate discontent will not pass until there is an invigorating autumn of freedom and equality. Nineteen sixty-three is not an end, but a beginning. Those who hope that the Negro needed to blow off steam and will now be content will have a rude awakening if the nation returns to business as usual. There will be neither rest nor tranquility in America until the Negro is granted his citizenship rights. The whirlwinds of revolt will continue to shake the foundations of our nation until the bright day of justice merges.

But there is something that I must say to my people who stand on the warm threshold which leads into the palace of justice. In the process of gaining our rightful place we must not be guilty of wrongful deed. Let us not seek to satisfy our thirst for freedom by drinking from the cup of bitterness and hatred. We must forever conduct our struggle on the high plane of dignity and discipline. We must not allow our creative protest to degenerate into physical violence. Again and again we must rise to the majestic heights of meeting physical force with soul force.

The marvelous new militancy which has engulfed the Negro community must not lead us to a distrust of all white people, for many of our white brothers, as evidenced by their presence here today, have come to realize that their destiny is tied up with our destiny and their freedom is inextricably bound to our freedom. We cannot walk alone.

And as we walk, we must make the pledge that we shall march ahead. We cannot turn back. There are those who are asking the devotees of civil rights, "When will you be satisfied?"

We can never be satisfied as long as the Negro is the victim of the unspeakable horrors of police brutality.

We can never be satisfied as long as our bodies, heavy with the fatigue of travel, cannot gain lodging in the motels of the highways and the hotels of the cities.

We cannot be satisfied as long as the Negro's basic mobility is from a smaller ghetto to a larger one.

We can never be satisfied as long as a Negro in Mississippi cannot vote and a Negro in New York believes he has nothing for which to vote.

No, no, we are not satisfied, and we will not be satisfied until justice rolls down like waters and righteousness like a mighty stream.

I am not unmindful that some of you have come here out of great trials and tribulations. Some of you have come fresh from narrow jail cells. Some of you have come from areas where your quest for freedom left you battered by the storms of persecution and staggered by the winds of police brutality. You have been the veterans of creative suffering. Continue to work with the faith that unearned suffering is redemptive.

Go back to Mississippi, go back to Alabama, go back to South Carolina, go back to Georgia, go back to Louisiana, go back to the slums and ghettos of our Northern cities, knowing that somehow this situation can and will be changed. Let us not wallow in the valley of despair.

I say to you today, my friends, that in spite of the difficulties and frustrations of the moment I still have a dream. It is a dream deeply rooted in the American dream.

I have a dream that one day this nation will rise up and live out the true meaning of its creed: "We hold these truths to be self-evident; that all men are created equal."

I have a dream that one day on the red hills of Georgia the sons of former slaves and the sons of former slave owners will be able to sit down together at the table of brotherhood.

I have a dream that one day even the state of Mississippi, a desert state sweltering with the heat of injustice and oppression, will be transformed into an oasis of freedom and justice.

I have a dream that my four little children will one day live in a nation where they will not be judged by the color of their skin but by the content of their character.

I have a dream today.

I have a dream that one day the state of Alabama, whose governor's lips are presently dripping with the words of interposition and nullification, will be transformed into a situation where little black boys and black girls will be able to join hands with little white boys and white girls and walk together as sisters and brothers.

I have a dream today.

I have a dream that one day every valley shall be exalted, every hill and mountain shall be made low, the rough places will be made plain, and the crooked places will be made straight, and the glory of the Lord shall be revealed, and all flesh shall see it together.

This is our hope. This is the faith with which I return to the South. With this faith we will be able to hew out of the mountain of despair a tone of hope. With this faith we will be able to transform the jangling discords of our nation into a beautiful symphony of brotherhood.

With this faith we will be able to work together, to pray together, to struggle together, to go to jail together, to stand up for freedom together, knowing that we will be free one day.

This will be the day when all of God's children will be able to sing with new meaning. "My country 'tis of thee, sweet land of liberty, of thee I sing. Land where my fathers died, land of the Pilgrims' pride, from every mountainside, let freedom ring."

And if America is to be a great nation, this must become true. So let freedom ring from the prodigious hilltops of New Hampshire. Let freedom ring from the mighty mountains of New York. Let freedom ring from the heightening Alleghenies of Pennsylvania! Let freedom ring from the snowcapped Rockies of Colorado! Let freedom ring from the curvaceous peaks of California! But not only that; let freedom ring from Stone Mountain of Georgia! Let freedom ring from Lookout Mountain of Tennessee! Let freedom ring from every hill and molehill of Mississippi. From every mountainside, let freedom ring.

When we let freedom ring, when we let it ring from every village and every hamlet, from every state and every city, we will be able to speed up that day when all of God's children, black men and white men, Jews and Gentiles, Protestants and Catholics, will be able to join hands and sing in the words of the old Negro spiritual, "Free at last! Free at last! Thank God Almighty, we are free at last!"

*   *   *

We are what we think.
All that we are arises with our thoughts.
With our thoughts we make the world.

The Buddha

*   *   *

I DREAM OF A HEALING HOUSE

PEGGY L. CHINN, a nurse and professor at the University of Colorado, is editor of Advances in Nursing Science *and acting editor of* Nursing Outlook. *These paragraphs closed a speech she delivered at Teachers College, New York (1988).*

I dreamed that I entered a place called a Healing House. . . . (p. 71)

This dream reflects what "health is wholeness" would mean in a situation for someone facing an "incurable" illness, what actions would arise from this meaning, and what transformations are needed in order to put this into action.

How do dreams come true? I begin to make this dream come true every time I act with conscious awareness, deliberately taking some experiential step in the direction of my dream. I begin to make it happen by explaining to myself and others what is happening as it happens. I begin to make it happen every time I recognize the imprisoning effect of our current system, to speak about circumstances that I see as preventing the dream from becoming reality, and work to change those circumstances. I begin to make my dream come true every time I talk with other nurses who can share the dream, and begin to create ways to work together from our diverse and varied perspectives. This is feminist praxis; it is also nursing praxis.

I believe that in the twenty-first century, people will look back on the health care system that existed in the twentieth century and see it as a medieval, barbaric form of care, much in the same way that we now view treatment of the mentally ill during the nineteenth century. I believe that the environments in which nurses will work to create health and wholeness for all will have little, if any, resemblance to today's working environment. I believe that out of our current crisis in nursing, we can incorporate the best of feminist insights to empower all women, and all nurses, to create the health-healing-wholeness environment of the twenty-first century.

ONLY AS MUCH AS I DREAM

DOROTHY JEAN NOVELLO was former dean of nursing at Villa Maria College, Erie, Pennsylvania, and was a former president of the National League for Nursing. This quotation was taken from a report she wrote just before she died in 1984. Did she mean this to be her epitaph, as well as a summons to those who survive?

> Only as high as I reach can I grow.
> Only as far as I seek can I go.
> Only as deep as I look can I see.
> Only as much as I dream can I be.

SOMETHING TO BELIEVE IN

SUE T. HEGYVARY is Professor and Dean, School of Nursing, University of Washington, Seattle.

A basic part of our culture is hope and believing in something beyond ourselves. Each fall, we nursing educators welcome a new group of students, full of hope and ideals. They see injustices that require correction; neglected people who deserve attention; illness that can be turned to health. They are determined to do something significant to make a difference in the lives of others. . . .

. . . nursing education and the world of practice tend to treat hope and idealism with amusement—"they will learn." Thoughts of improving the current status quo belong to Don Quixote and others who spend their lives charging windmills. As a result, we have a population of nurses who are worn down and worn out by disillusionment. Many of those same dreamers of yesterday now resist ideals, convinced that today's reality is tomorrow's necessity. . . .

Having something to believe in doesn't mean naively recycling the noble ideals of yesterday. Planning for the future requires us to define our hopes and dreams, weigh them against the current facts, and take the necessary calculated risks to see if ideals and goals can be made real. (p. 76)

> Weighing, choosing, risk-taking, independence, courage, strategy, timing are embedded throughout the literature about making a difference, as illustrated in the following selections.

The Bravest

But the bravest are surely those who have the clearest vision of what is before them, glory and danger alike, and yet notwithstanding go out to meet it.

> Thucydides, Peloponnesian War, Book II,
> (Funeral Oration of Pericles), section 40

THE ROAD NOT TAKEN

ROBERT FROST (1874–1963) has long been recognized as one of America's greatest and most widely read poets. Several of his books of poetry won Pulitzer prizes. He taught at Amherst, Harvard, Dartmouth, and the University of Michigan.

Two roads diverged in a yellow wood,
And sorry I could not travel both
And be one traveler, long I stood
And looked down one as far as I could
To where it bent in the undergrowth;

Then took the other, as just as fair,
And having perhaps the better claim,
Because it was grassy and wanted wear;
Though as for that, the passing there
Had worn them really about the same,

And both that morning equally lay
In leaves no step had trodden black.
Oh, I kept the first for another day!
Yet knowing how way leads on to way,
I doubted if I should ever come back.

I shall be telling this with a sigh
Somewhere ages and ages hence:
Two roads diverged in a wood, and I—
I took the one less traveled by,
And that has made all the difference. (p. 105)

MARKINGS

DAG HJALMAR AGNE CARL HAMMARSKJOLD (1905–1961) was awarded the 1961 Nobel Peace Prize posthumously for his peace-keeping efforts in Suez, Lebanon, and the Congo. A political leader in his native Sweden, he served as secretary-general of the United Nations from 1953 until his death in a plane crash in 1961. This excerpt is from his book, Markings.

It is more important to be aware of the grounds for your own behavior than to understand the motives of another.

The other's "face" is more important than your own. If, while pleading another's cause, you are at the same time seeking something for yourself, you cannot hope to succeed.

You can only hope to find a lasting solution to a conflict if you have learned to see the other objectively, but, at the same time, to experience his difficulties subjectively.

The man who "likes people" disposes once and for all of the man who despises them.

All first hand experience is valuable, and he who has given up looking for it will one day find—that he lacks what he needs: a closed mind is a weakness, and he who approaches persons or painting or poetry without the youthful ambition to learn a new language and so gain access to someone else's perspective on life, let him beware.

A successful lie is doubly a lie, an error which has to be corrected is a heavier burden than truth: only an uncompromising "honesty" can reach the bedrock of decency which you should always expect to find, even under deep layers of evil.

Diplomatic "finesse" must never be another word for fear of being unpopular: that is to seek the appearance of influence at the cost of its reality. (p. 114)

*   *   *

There is nothing more difficult to take in hand, more perilous to conduct or more uncertain in its success, than to take the lead in the introduction of a new order of things, because the innovator has for enemies all those who have done well under the old system, and lukewarm defenders in those who may do well under the new.

Niccolo Machiavelli (1469–1527), The Prince

When I entered into service here, I determined that, happen what would, I never would intrigue among the Committee. Now I perceive that I do all my business by intrigue. I propose in private to A, B, or C the resolution I think A, B, or C most capable of carrying in Committee, and then leave it to them, and I always win. (p. 53)

Florence Nightingale

A TIME TO DECIDE

DENISE A. NIEMIRA, a physician from Wichita Falls, Texas, wrote this article that appeared in the "A Piece of My Mind" column in a 1982 Journal of the American Medical Association.

I lifted from her arms the body that I first had laid there just 20 months before. Once the official pronouncer of birth, I was now the official pronouncer of death, dismantling the living pieta—the sorrowful mother cradling her dead son.

A few days before, Julie and I stood outside my office. She held Christopher, limp and whimpering, in her arms. It was the day the medical center had prearranged for Christopher's chemotherapy. I held the vial of asparaginase. As their family physician, I would administer the injection as I had before, to save them an 80-mile trip to the oncology clinic.

But this visit was like none of the others. If Julie had sensed this difference when she scheduled Christopher's appointment outside routine office hours, she did not voice her fears over the phone. I myself had no forewarning of any new problems when I went to meet the family in my office parking lot and accepted the vial of asparaginase they handed me. Nothing was unusual about our conversation. But somewhere in the short distance between parking lot and office, I realized something was indeed different. Perhaps it was Julie's hesitancy to follow me in, or the especially protective way in which she held her son. Before we reached the building, she explored: "Is it really necessary to give him this shot?"

I stopped short and looked at mother and child, taking stock of just how sick Christopher was. The ecchymoses that had previously dotted his pale body now covered it, and he had gone from listless to limp. My mind raced over the details of his illness: the B-cell leukemia, the central nervous system involvement, the short remission, the persisting relapse. Christopher's last dose of chemotherapy had been administered at the medical center. Perhaps the source of Julie's question could be traced to the events of that last visit.

I had not heard recently from either of Christopher's pediatric oncologists. I knew the older one, who usually managed Christopher's case, as a relentless warrior in the struggle against childhood leukemia who was unlikely to discontinue therapy even at the end. I knew his younger partner was a softer, more "humanistic" man who could allow for other options in the face of inevitable death.

When I asked Julie about the visit, she recounted her conversation with the younger physician. "He said that Christopher would probably die from his illness and that it was up to us whether to continue chemotherapy. I don't want Christopher to die," she continued, sobbing, "but I don't see how the medicine's helping and I don't want him to be in pain."

She mentioned Christopher's fever, and I realized then that there was more than a chemotherapy decision at stake. "Julie," I began, "did the doctor tell you how leukemic children die?"

Julie's eyes met mine, the eyes of a naturally bright young woman who was also a product of the culture of a poor, rural area. My mind searched hurriedly for the "right" phrases, phrases that would help her understand, words that might help to soften the grim news: "bleeding because of the low number of platelets that help blood to clot . . ." "overwhelming infection because of the low number of white cells that help fight germs . . . ." Somehow the words came, ending with my simple statement, "Christopher may be dying now."

We talked about treatment, no longer asparaginase but hospitalization, diagnostic testing, IV antibiotics, and other supportive therapy. We also talked about no treatment. Julie did not want to take Christopher to the medical center or even to our local hospital. She sobbed again, "I don't want Christopher to die, but if he's going to die, I wanted it to be at home. I don't want him to have any more pain when it isn't going to help." Julie's husband concurred. As I looked at Christopher lying in her arms, I felt this was the right choice. On the slim chance that Christopher had a minor infection, I wrote a prescription for oral antibiotics and sent him home with his parents.

Afterward I telephoned the oncologists' office to inform them about Christopher's condition and our decision. The younger partner, who was on call, answered. He remembered his discussion with Julie. "The prognosis was bad from the start," he said. "I understand your decision and I'm available to help if you should need it."

Christopher stayed at home. He died after several days. Hospice nurses helped with his care, injecting morphine when even the gentle touch of caring hands caused him pain. The pediatric intern from the oncology clinic drove 90 miles on his weekend off to say good-bye to Christopher and also to observe this death outside a medical institution.

Christopher died in his wooden crib, in a log cabin that his family called home. There were no tubes, no wires, no lines to disconnect as I removed him, lifeless, from his mother's arms. Christopher died the victim of his disease, not the victim of medical interventions. He had received conventional treatment, but when it failed, his parents could say "Enough is enough" and take him home to die.

Christopher might have lived longer; he might have died more slowly, if we had made another decision that day. I will never know.

Other physicians might have framed the options differently; other parents might have chosen another course of action. When a life is hanging in the balance, there is no easy decision.

Christopher was the first but not the only child whose body I lifted from his mother's at birth and again at his death. Julie and her husband were not the only parents with whom I agonized over options and choices, learning that there is no right way but that there is a way that feels right.

When I think now of Christopher as I last saw him, lying in his mother's arms, I am reminded of the passage in Ecclesiastes: "To every thing there is a season, and a time to every purpose under the heaven. A time to be born, and a time to die."

Sometimes, between the two, there is another time—a time to decide. (p. 1913)

FOR EVERYTHING ITS SEASON

For everything its season, and for every activity under
heaven its time:
    a time to be born and a time to die;
    a time to plant and a time to uproot;
    a time to kill and a time to heal;
    a time to break down and a time to build up;
    a time to weep and a time to laugh;
    a time for mourning and a time for dancing;
    a time to scatter stones and a time to gather them;
    a time to embrace and a time to abstain from
        embracing;
    a time to seek and a time to lose;
    a time to keep and a time to discard;
    a time to tear and a time to mend;
    a time for silence and a time for speech;
    a time to love and a time to hate;
    a time for war and a time for peace.

Ecclesiastes, 2, 3.

Letters to the editor, as a literary form, have lent themselves well to dispensing accolades for unsung heroes. Thus we read next about nurses who make a difference, just some of the millions of nurses around the world who carry out daily both a collective and an individual mission.

LETTER TO THE EDITOR

B.T. COLLINS (1934–1993) was a veteran of the Vietnam War, vice-president of a securities firm in Sacramento, CA, and a California State Assemblyman. This letter appeared in the California Nursing Review *(1988).*

Recently, I received your magazine from a friend of mine. . . . I was particularly moved by the cover story "Vietnam—A Legacy of Healing." I write not only to commend you for publishing the article but also in the hope that perhaps my letter will reach any former Vietnam nurse in your readership. I would especially like to talk to those who have any doubts similar to those expressed in the article, who wondered if it was right for them to save us.

First of all, that answer is unfathomable. So don't even trouble yourself by asking the question. My company commander was shot in the head and in the legs on his 27th birthday, 1967. He lived for 17 years and in October of 1984 I buried him. He lived with literally half a brain and as a quadriplegic. He probably had an IQ of about 83.

However, he married and ended up having a tremendous effect on other people's lives, including mine. For those of you who are interested, you can see him on November 23rd when they rebroadcast the Kennedy funeral. He is the 1st Lt. in charge of President Kennedy's body who is standing at the rear of the casket.

I was blown up by my own hand grenade in June of 1967 during my second tour in a swamp in the Lon Toan Secret Zone in the Mekong Delta.

When I arrived at the Third Surgical Hospital at Dong Tam, I was filthy, bearded, covered with jungle sores and red ants. I was missing an arm and my legs were shattered. My blood pressure was 45 over nothing, my Ph was 6.7 and I was about to undergo two cardiac arrests. There were very few American casualties that night. I guess they were able to take this barely recognizable Green Beret and put him on the table where the nurses and the doctors started to work immediately. They took my leg above the knee, gave me 39 pints of blood and my life in return.

Twenty-two months, 29 operations, and seven military hospitals later, I left the army and began an entirely new career. From 1979 to 1981, I ran the largest youth employment program in the United States, the California Conservation Corps. It is now being emulated by 39 other states and 15 other countries. It has affected the lives of thousands of young people and hopefully has instilled in them a work ethic and the notion that you must give back to society instead of taking from it.

There are those in the press and in government who say I made a difference. But I know who really made a difference and it was those 19-to 20-year-old nurses who in 1967 held on to my one remaining hand and got me to hang on. Unless you've been there, you will never have any idea what their gentleness, their strength, their perfume, their beautiful skin, their cleanliness meant to us. You simply will never have any idea.

Even in the States where we had clean sheets, they were there to somehow make the dressing changes just a little more tolerable. They were there when we woke up screaming in the OR. They were there when our parents and our girls came to visit us for the first time. They were there when we took our first steps. They were there when we got the reality checks that happened when we left the hospital to face the uncaring and unsympathetic public. Always, they were just there. They covered for us when we were AWOL. They simply made a difference.

So if I am reaching any of you out there, I just want you to know one thing. Our lives were irrevocably changed by the presence of those military nurses. You did something that no one else could do. And I swear to you that we will never ever ever forget you.

*   *   *

Security is mostly superstition. It does not exist in nature, nor do the children of men as a whole experience it. Avoiding danger is no safer in the long run than outright exposure. Life is either a daring adventure, or nothing.

Helen Keller, *The Open Door,* 1957

XI

ON WRITING

*I*f we had to say what writing is, we would define it essentially as an act of courage

Cynthia Ozick, *New York Times,* 1983

Nurses of the world, do write!

On Nursing: A Literary Celebration has presented selections—both classical and contemporary, general and professional—illustrating how we can benefit from literature of all forms. While it is an important first step to appreciate literature, it is quite another step to create literature. Thus, as we near the end of this volume, we are left with the questions: "Why should we write?" and "How and what could we add to this literature?" This final chapter touches upon these questions.

As nurses, we should write to enrich our lives, our practice, and our profession. We should write to explore and communicate our experiences. We should write as a means of burnishing our image and bolstering our self-concept as well-educated, well-rounded persons. We should write to expand our repertoires and our horizons as professionals.

Nursing has a special role and privilege in society and health care that surfaces throughout these pages. That role and privilege give us much to convey to nurses and other health professionals about our calling and our craft. As to the people we serve, we, and only we, can tell nursing's true story to the public—the story of our heritage and of our health care beliefs, goals, and contributions. Most of all, we should write because we have something to say that needs to be said. And we need to say it in ways that capture the attention and respect of readers and, in so doing, incite them to join us in "making a difference."

How well have we done getting our message across to the world at large? Can we do better? All nurses know personally and painfully that we suffer from an image problem. But, for a more objective opinion we might read Suzanne Gordon, author of *Prisoner of Men's Dreams,* who sums it up this way:

> *Ironically, whenever popular culture deals with the medical system, the important role of nursing is almost always trivialized or ignored altogether. On the other hand, the depiction of physicians . . . has always been far more favorable and equally unrealistic. On TV and in movies, physicians linger devotedly at their patients' bedsides and show interest in the intimate details of their lives. Nurses, meanwhile, make an occasional bedside appearance to take a temperature or monitor a heartbeat. . . .*
>
> *The same imbalance is evident in bookstores. Numerous mass market books chart the intricacies of medical education and health care and describe the experiences of individual physicians. Nursing books, however, have been ghettoized in the textbook departments of academic publishers; as a result, the public rarely glimpses nursing's serious contributions to health care. And most news stories about health care totally ignore the fact that nurses are also health care experts and legitimate sources for insight, analysis, comment, and information. (p. 145)*

We must make nursing visible in all its power and glory. To the growing and esteemed ranks of nurse practitioners, nurse educators, nurse administrators, nurse researchers, and nurse lawyers, we must add increasing numbers of nurse writers. Each of us is a candidate, because to be a nurse writer is not to exclude other roles, but to draw upon, augment, and enhance those "practice" dimensions. We must enlarge and incorporate within our profession the culture of creative communication merged with our dominant culture of dedicated service.

What is the base from which we can launch such a campaign? Norman Cousins, cited several times in this volume, has compared writers and physicians in an article for a medical journal (Cousins, 1982). We might argue that many of his observations about the similarities and differences apply equally to our situation. For example, couldn't it be said that nurses and writers deal with health and disease—nurses with the health and ills of persons, writers with the health and ills of society? Wouldn't we agree that writers help to create change and nurses often deal with the effects of it? Isn't it the case that, as much as we may shun the spoken reality, nurses have direct power over people; writers have the power to create or recreate people. Surely we resonate to Cousins' assertion that anecdotal, "nonverifiable" results are anathema to clinical scientists; yet anecdotes that shed light on human behavior are the raw materials "stalked" and savored by writers, to whom no data are "soft." And isn't it true that, in the final analysis, our greatest strength as nurses may be in our artistry, the balancing of tangibles with intangibles, a realization to which our professional literature is now reawakening? All in all, it does seem that, despite the contrasts, common ground spans the two cultures of nursing and writing.

What does it take to be a writer? The qualities required to create literature are *inspiration, artistry, skill,* and *life experiences.*

Literature begins with the *inspiration* to put together words that trace a line of history or thought, tell a story, or capture a feeling—all of this for one's own satisfaction as well as to interact with others. The writer uses words for creative expression, just as the sculptor and artist use the visual forms of shape and color and texture.

The *artistry* in writing is in recognizing that the printed page takes on sound as well as meaning as its words are picked up by the mind and the senses of the reader, and in balancing and fine-tuning these aspects to achieve the sensations and understandings intended. Words written have a visual, auditory, cognitive, and affective impact, determined by how they are selected and ordered and presented. And it is often the smallest detail, the shaded nuance, the subtlest synchrony, the softest touch brushed across the text that makes the difference between distinguished and undistinguished writing and imprints our personal stamp upon the page.

The writer who composes literature and the reader who appreciates literature similarly understand that language, at its most magnificent, walks us down a tortured path of reasoning, orchestrates sounds and rhythms within the inner ear, paints pictures for the unseeing eye, awakens remembered smells and tastes, and stirs a tide of emotions.

As would be expected, the best writers have said this best. Their feeling for words and language lights the following passages by Eudora Welty, David Noonan, and Anne Sexton. As we read, the mind quickens; the senses are alert.

One Writer's Beginnings

Eudora Welty is a Southern writer of short stories whose work has been honored by the Pulitzer Prize, the American Book Award for Fiction, and the Gold Medal for the Novel, bestowed by the American Academy and Institute of Arts and Letters for her entire work in fiction. She still lives in her father's house in Jackson, Mississippi, the town of her birth. The following selection is taken from her 1984 work, One Writer's Beginnings.

In my sensory education I include my physical awareness of the *word.* Of a certain word, that is; the connection it has with what it stands for. At around age six, perhaps, I was standing by myself in our front yard waiting for supper, just at that hour in a late summer day when the sun is already below the horizon and the risen full moon in the visible sky stops being chalky and begins to take on light. There comes the moment, and I saw it then, when the moon goes from flat to round. For the first time it met my eyes as a globe. The word "moon" came into my mouth as though fed to me out of a silver spoon. Held in my mouth the moon became a word. It had the roundness of a Concord grape Grandpa took off his vine and gave me to suck out of its skin and swallow whole, in Ohio. (p. 10)

LANGUAGE

DAVID NOONAN

Think about language, in the variety of its forms. The precise line of it that connects two people in serious conversation, each word selected with care, inflections modulated for accuracy. The lone point of it in the author's room at the moment of creation, when the words and sentences arrive as though they have come from some other place. The relaxed web of it at a party, language trailing about the room, supple and unpredictable, free of scrutiny and planning, in the service of simple human pleasure, language as talk, as jokes told, and secrets whispered. The murmuring bowl of it that fills stadiums and arenas when the action is slow, the low rumble of ten thousand quiet conversations, and the roaring wall of it that erupts with a score. The surprising beam of it that lights the world when the poet puts just the right words in just the right places. The slumbering mass of it stacked in the libraries, waiting to be read, language as literary enterprise, bound to outlive the writers. The silent bond of it that joins reader and book. The sudden rip of it that is a scream for help. The murderer's mumbled confession, the first-grader's correct answer, the lover's lie, the priest's blessing, the condemned man's last words, the son's promise, the professor's lecture, the madman's ranting, the President's speech, the bad novel, the dead letter, the good novel, the memo, the prayer, the chant, the baby's first coherent syllable.

There is no end to the list. Language engulfs us, swirls about us; like our bubble of oxygen, it envelops the planet. We spin it out endlessly and it comes back to us endlessly. Language is the prime mechanism for the organization and expression of the workings of the human mind, it is the skill that enables us to engage in the limitless complexities of human life, and it is the means by which we chronicle that life. Language is an elaborate, dynamic, living thing.

And in most people it originates on the left side of the brain, in a few patches of cortex that, combined, are about the size of a postcard. (pp. 158–159)

WORDS

ANNE SEXTON's The Complete Poems, *published in 1981, included this selection.*

Be careful of words,
even the miraculous ones.
For the miraculous we do our best,
sometimes they swarm like insects
and leave not a sting but a kiss.
They can be as good as fingers.
They can be as trusty as the rock
you stick your bottom on.
But they can be both daisies and bruises.

Yet I am in love with words.
They are doves falling out of the ceiling.
They are six holy oranges sitting in my lap.
They are the trees, the legs of summer,
and the sun, its passionate face.

Yet often they fail me.
I have so much I want to say,
so many stories, images, proverbs, etc.
But the words aren't good enough,
the wrong ones kiss me.
Sometimes I fly like an eagle
but with the wings of a wren.

But I try to take care
and be gentle to them.
Words and eggs must be handled with care.
Once broken they are impossible
things to repair. (p. 463)

The *craft* of writing, a third quality necessary to creating literature, encompasses a broad range of skills from the self-discipline
of the task to the mechanics and structure of the composition
and, eventually, to negotiating the world of publishing. These
skills can be learned through courses and seminars and books on
literature and creative writing, through supervised practice, and
through association with published writers.

How do successful writers feel about their work, their craft? A
small sample of those emotions can be felt in the following brief
selections in which the solitude, labor, discipline, and frustration—all powered by the engine of an overwhelming urge to
write—are described by experienced authors.

WORKING

*ALICE KOLLER earned her doctorate in philosophy at Harvard,
and has lived in New England most of her life. She is the author
of* An Unknown Woman *and* The Stations of Solitude *from
which this excerpt is taken.*

I write my thinking. I think by writing. I persist in the belief that I
can articulate whatever I think about. Because I persist, I can. Because I know how, I can. By the words I choose, by their sound
and sequence and significance, I shape for you new eyes, new
ears, a new mind, so that you, reading, listening, say, "Yes, that's
what I mean (or see, or think, or hear)." I write what I mean, what
I understand, what I know. This is my work.

It is a peculiar kind of work, writing one's thinking. It is not writing
fiction, or poetry, or criticism, or history, or plays. It is not even
autobiography. It is not reportage, or commentary on current
events. It is not instruction in some economically useful skill. It
is not homily. Several philosophers, all men, all secure in their
tenured positions at major universities, tell me (indeed, they insist) that it is not philosophy, but they are the same people who let
me hang in the wind. Members of English departments are uncomfortable (because it is not fiction or poetry or . . .). Essays, perhaps? Yes, I essay to write my thinking. I am a philosopher

studying my own mind. And when I look outward at the natural world, I essay to write my seeing and hearing and touching. (p. 41)

DARING DREAMER

CARLOS FUENTES, Mexico's pre-eminent novelist, author of The Old Gringo *and* The Death of Artemis Cruz, *is quoted in an article by interviewer Guy Garcia for* Time *(June 1992).*

I think there are things that deserve to be said. . . . I am not a professional rebel or enfant terrible. Yet . . . in a way [controversy] goes with the territory. . . because it is not natural to write. We are created to run and hunt and swim and make love but not to sit hunched with a piece of paper and some ink scribbling hieroglyphs. And when we do it, it is an act of rebellion against God himself, who did not design us to do that. So I've always said the writer in a way is the brother of Lucifer—he is rebellious and arrogant and condemned, but he is having a good time. . . . Until the fires start burning! (p. 78)

WRITING A BOOK

GEORGE ORWELL (1903–1950) was the pen name of Eric Blair, British political writer and author of Animal Farm *and* 1984.

Writing a book is a horrible, exhausting struggle, like a long bout of some painful illness. One would never undertake such a thing if one were not driven by some demon whom one can neither resist nor understand. For all one knows that demon is simply the same instinct that makes a baby squall for attention. And yet it is also true that one can write nothing readable unless one constantly struggles to efface one's personality. Good prose is like a windowpane.

Writing Is Writing

E. L. Doctorow is an American novelist who often intertwines actual historical figures and events with fictional characters, as in the bestselling novel Ragtime.

Planning to write is not writing. Outlining a book is not writing. Researching is not writing. Talking to people about what you're doing, none of that is writing. Writing is writing.

Inspiration, skill, and artistry. To these three essentials nurse writers can add our fourth and greatest asset—our vast and unique storehouse of *life experience*. It is not hyperbole to boast that no writer of highest stature has ever enjoyed richer opportunities to observe human nature and human pathos than *every* nurse. Day after day and for sustained intervals we see life at its most intimate, most exposed, most vulnerable, and most heroic. So, to the question, "What do we have to add to the literature?" the answer is "Our experiences and the lessons we have learned from them." We have magnificent stories to tell and powerful observations to make and thoughts to share.

The manner in which we tell our stories, the philosophy underlying our narration, the language and metaphors we use, if picked up and passed along, have the power to change people's views of their health and eventually influence public policy on health care.

There is also a body of literature on the value of storytelling and the power of the words and the images they evoke. Various purposes served by storytelling and the might of the metaphor are the subjects of the several pieces presented below.

The Healing Art

Clarissa Pinkola Estes is a senior Jungian analyst with more than two decades of practice and teaching experience. An award-winning author, she is a cantadora and artist-in-residence for the state of Colorado. Her first book, Women Who Run with the Wolves: Myths and Stories of the Wild Woman Archetype

(1992), became an almost instant bestseller, from which the following excerpt was taken.

Storytelling is bringing up, hauling up; it is not an idle practice. Though there are story trades, wherein two people exchange stories as a gift to one another, for the most part they have come to know each other well; they have developed, if they are not born to it, a kinship relationship. And this is as it should be.

Although some use stories as entertainment alone, tales are, in their oldest sense, a healing art. Some are called to this healing art, and the best, to my lights, are those who have lain with the story and found all its matching parts inside themselves and at depth. . . . In the best tellers I know, the stories grow out of their lives like roots grow a tree. The stories have grown *them,* grown them into who they are.

WITHOUT STORIES

CAROL CHRIST is a feminist author who emphasizes the importance of stories as a way of knowing and as an essential means of passing on that understanding to future generations. Her books include Reflections on a Journey to the Goddess *and* Diving Deep and Surfacing: Women Writers on Spiritual Quest, *from which this passage is taken.*

Without stories there is no articulation of experience. Without stories a woman is lost when she comes to make the important decisions in her life. She does not learn to value her struggles, to celebrate her strengths, to comprehend her pain. Without stories she is alienated from the deeper experiences of self and world that have been called spiritual or religious. (p. 1)

MY MOTHER'S STORIES

HIROKO B. YAMANO is the daughter of a Japanese American woman interred during World War II. The following poem was written for Bettina Aptheker's class on feminism and reprinted in her Tapestries of Life.

> I don't want to tell her my stories
> I am old.
> I don't remember.
> My stories were of long time ago.
> I locked my stories in a box.
> I buried the key.
>
> My daughter wants my stories.
> Her soul is too restless.
> I can't keep her quiet.
> She wants to know about my past,
> about the old,
> about something that is gone.
>
> I don't want her to come home.
> She's here.
> She waits endlessly,
> in my garden
> > in my dreams
> > for my answers.
> > I know
> > someday
> > she'll be knocking
> > at my grave
> > she'll stand there
> > wanting my stories
>
> I can only tell her,
> > I am old
> > I don't remember
> > My stories were of long time ago.
> > I locked my stories in a box.
> > I buried the key.
> > > Now you must go. (pp. 31–32)

FIGHTING THE ENEMY AND OTHER FINAL CHAPTERS: PAYING THE PRICE OF OUR STORIES

JUDITH WILSON ROSS is with the Center for Bioethics, St. Joseph's Health System, Orange, California. These excerpts are from a presentation made at the West Coast Hastings Center 20th Anniversary Celebration in San Francisco, 1989.

The controlling metaphor for American medicine is war and the controlling narrative for American health care is that immortality is achievable (a) because disease is external, (b) because the body is essentially a machine and thus repairable and reconstructible, (c) because human destiny is to control nature, and (d) because death is failure (the patient's, the physician's, or both). The controlling narrative for individuals is that they are the authors of their lives.

Our favorite medical story is called "Fighting the Enemy." This story is intertwined with another story called "Fixing Machines." We also have a story (a metaphor within a metaphor) called "Writing Our Life." This story assumes that we can control every aspect of our lives, including how and even whether we die (the ultimate in personal control). Writing Our Life is closely related to Fighting the Enemy. That is, if we are successful in Writing Our Life, then we will be successful when disease threatens in Fighting the Enemy because Writing Our Life assumes we are in control. If we lose at Fighting, the implication is that we have also failed at Writing. The public movement to obtain Death with Dignity (a sub-story of Writing Our Life) is actually an attempt to combine Writing Our Life with Fighting the Enemy for, when losing to disease becomes inevitable, control can be retained by shifting the focus of control.

These are the stories that have no room for less medical treatment. Although novelists themselves often talk about how, when writing, their characters take over (suggesting that being an author is not really characterized by total control), the narrative of Writing Our Lives suggests otherwise: Writing is about Being in Control. If we are to be the authors of our lives, we must stave off disease and, ultimately, death, because they impair our ability to author. That is, since disease is seen as an abnormal state that comes to us from outside ourselves, disease itself is evidence of our failure to be in control. To be sick indicates an (at least temporary) victory for the enemy. Thus, the appearance of disease indicates a loss of control (this is simply a variation on disease as sin, a much older metaphor). Furthermore, the very process of disease imposes a further reduction in our ability to control our destiny because of physical and perhaps emotional/mental impairment.

Our version of Writing Our Lives implies a kind of Manichean world in which there is a constant battle between that which would try to control us and that which we try to control. Disease belongs to the external world, the world of nature, and is decidedly "not us." (Think of Ronald Reagan who explained after his surgery that he didn't have cancer: that there was something inside of him that had cancer in it and *that* is what was removed.) Because disease is "not us," we need total access to whatever medical science has in order to exert or re-exert control over the enemy. Indeed, medical technology is a publicly funded extension of self—the weapons and tools designed to regain control.

If this is an accurate portrayal of the health care story in which most Americans are living, then it is clear why denial of potentially beneficial medical treatment seems impossible, unthinkable, and, if it happens, a profound injustice. If we need to fight the enemy in order to maintain our control so that we can be the authors of our lives, we need the resources to conduct the war properly. In time of war, the needs of war take priority. You do not ration goods for those on the battle line. It is those at home—the healthy—who will have to make do with less. Thus, some argue that, if medical care requires an increasing proportion of our gross national product, so be it. It is surely ironic, however, that the military budget is most often proposed as the site for extracting additional medical care funds. By going to defense, we rob war to pay for war.

Now, it would be one kind of problem if the public espoused this narrative and the medical world espoused some other narrative (for example, "Healing the Patient"). If different narratives were at work, tensions between patient and physician would be extraordinary. However, the medical world is at least as enthusiastic about Fighting the Enemy as is the public. For example, Janssen Pharmaceutics tells me that when I am tired out from fighting allergies 24 hours a day, my doctor can help me fight back because he is in control of allergy weapons that work day and night, and with his help, I can win! . . . Medical advertising, medical writing, and medical vocabulary are all filled with evidence of medicine's devotion to the war against disease. . . .

If patient and physician are unsuccessful in Fighting the Enemy, the result is Death. Many writers have delineated how, for the physician, Death is Failure. Early 20th century novelist-physician S. Weir Mitchell has a physician-protagonist who proclaims: "What I personally hate is defeat, by death, by incurable ailments."[1] Barbara Koenig's late 20th century housestaff seem to share this view. Contemplating a liver transplant for a desperately ill patient, the housestaff see the action as "a potential therapeutic solution to an otherwise insurmountable problem—the death of a patient." . . . Koenig describes the housestaff's pursuit of treatment as a ritual commitment: "medical interventions [are] offered as 'gifts of life' . . . [that] represent medicine's battle with death: It is the fight itself that becomes important." . . . When the physicians have no more "tricks," the patient must be acknowledged as dying: "Dying," again to quote Koenig, "becomes a cultural metaphor which symbolizes treatment failure."

If Death is problematic for the physician, it is even more so for the patient ensconced in this narrative. If the patient's condition fails to improve, medical metaphor often attribute the responsibility for this to the patient: thus, for example, the patient "fails chemotherapy." Chemotherapy does not fail the patient. Nor does the physician fail the patient. "There is nothing I can do," is not something one is likely to hear frequently in the hospital, since there is almost always something more that the physician can do. However, if that something doesn't help, responsibility for losing the fight begins to fall upon the patient who, technologically powerless, then has only two choices in the Writing Our Lives/ Fighting the Enemy story. First, the patient can turn to other modes of therapy, non-standard modes that may be able to defeat the enemy by using a different battle strategy. Second, the patient can begin to work on the end of the story; that is, to author the end of his/her life. It is at this point of the story that the public movements for active euthanasia, assisted suicide, and death with dignity have focused their work. Although they often present themselves as a counter movement, they are firmly in the story, disagreeing only about how the story is to be written, not about whether it is a story that is being written. They think it is time to end the story, but not because no more treatment is possible. It is because they can't have more treatment and still remain in control of their story. Further treatment means that they risk losing their authorship and the end of their life will then be written by someone else. In the hospital, as in Hollywood, no director (to change the metaphor slightly) wants to let somebody else have final cut.

If the metaphor/narratives of Fighting the Enemy and Writing Our Lives do not permit consideration of less treatment, are there other metaphor/narratives that offer alternatives to our financing/access crisis? . . .

What might such a narrative be like? And how might it conflict with our current narrative? The Canadian philosopher Michael Ignatieff, in a review essay written last year, suggests that a more useful narrative would be one based on stoicism. (It is probably not accidental that this view comes from one living in England.) He opines that "cultures that live by the values of self-realization and self-mastery are not especially good at dying, at submitting to those experiences where freedom ends and biological fate begins." It would seem that the American story does not even acknowledge that there is such a thing as biological fate. Stoicism, in combination with an "ironic relationship" to our view of selfhood would provide a sharp contrast, Ignatieff says, to

> the metaphor that leads us to regard our life as a narrative that
> we compose as we go along, with a beginning, a middle, and
> an end. This is a metaphor that convinces us that we are the
> makers of our lives, when, in fact, chance and contingency and

*the dull determination of living all combine to push our lives
into sequences we neither desire nor intend. To accept death is
to accept much more than that we do not write the end of the
story; it is also to appreciate that we don't write much of the
beginning or the middle either.*

Ignatieff offers one alternative that would certainly allow the
prospect of specific rationing as long as limitations were not totally arbitrary. Robert Lifton offers another in his exploration of
Death as Continuity: in this story, life is understood as offering
continuity despite death, continuity through offspring, through
creative works, through spiritual modes, and through personal
transcendence. Lifton attempts to circumvent the problem of
death as an end to personal control by creating a different understanding of death as a point in which personal control is transformed into personal continuity.

Moving to Heaven still offers a viable narrative for those who
have available to them the prospect of an after life (and one oncologist has told me that he has observed a distinct difference
between Jews with terminal cancer and Catholics with terminal
cancer, a difference that he attributed to their different understandings of an after life).

Death as Natural Event is a story in the making given the recent
enthusiasm for things natural in this culture. Indeed, the power of
contemporary medicine's single most important image, the body
attached to and kept alive by machines, with "tubes attached
everywhere," is largely a function of the unnaturalness of the image. To be reduced to the status of appendage to a machine is
even worse than being treated as a machine!

Childbirth is one form of medical care that has been significantly
altered by appeals to Nature and the Natural. However, one
should not underestimate the force of dominant cultural narratives considering that medicine has countered the natural childbirth movement by making not only childbirth but reproduction
itself increasingly technology dependent. The hospice movement
is certainly positioned to incorporate appeals to Death as Natural
Event as an important aspect of its own narrative. . . .

Finally, Healing the Patient (as opposed to Curing the Disease) offers a very different understanding of medicine. This story flourishes in the humanistic medical movement and, apparently somewhat independently, in the holistic medicine movement, a movement organized initially by patients. Healing the Patient is a narrative that does not necessarily accept direct rationing, but would be amenable to less dependence upon medical technology and perhaps to implicit rationing and could accept less medical treatment generally. Such a story would necessarily include a very different understanding of the relationship between body and mind.

Whatever story we are to use, death would continue to require appropriate social rituals. Philip Aries has described several distinct historical views of death and their accompanying rituals: death as an impersonal event, in which the person understood that his time had come and simply stopped his activities, lay down, crossed his arms, and awaited death; death as a personal event in which the awareness of impending death necessitated a personal accounting of one's life; and death as a familial event, in which death required a resolution of personal relationships. Each of these understandings gives the dying person a specific role and thus a structure for action. The physician, sharing this understanding of the patient's duties, could use his/her skills to help their patient fulfill their role.

In our world, the dying patient has a very peculiar role: it is *not to die*. "Don't crump out on me!" the physician yells in frustration and fear. The physician's job is to help the patient not to die by providing all possible treatment. If we are to hope that physicians and patients can move into a different story, it must include different roles for both dying person and health care professional. One cannot remove the obligation—the compulsion, even—to treat that Fighting the Enemy imposes unless it is replaced by some other meaningful ritual.

The critical factor in our story of disease is, of course, death. Joseph Campbell has suggested that primitive mythology offers two contrasting views of Death. The first, found "among the hunting tribes whose life style is based on the art of killing and who live in a world of animals that kill and are killed. [Here] all death is a consequence of violence and is generally ascribed not to the natural destiny of temporal beings but to magic. Magic is employed both to defend against it and to deliver it to others." . . . The contrasting view, that of the "planting folk," is that "death is a natural phase of life, comparable to the moment of the planting of the seed, for rebirth." . . . In this second narrative, life and death constitute a cycle, and the task for the living is to find ways of carrying the dead forward in their own lives, thereby providing continuity. Clearly our culture is captured by the former view. The price of America's own version of that story, however, is more magic and more powerful magic; i.e., ever increasing medical costs. That is the story we are now paying for.

A call to rationing must inevitably come up against the demand—indeed the need—for more magic. It is only by finding our connections with a different story, a different mythology, that this conflict can be resolved. The most important purpose of mythology, it has been said, is to carry the individual from old age to death. Our stories don't do this well, but there are other stories available to us. It is possible that change is already brewing in our culture. Responses to AIDS, for example, have certainly shown us the strength of the impulse to fight disease. But there are other responses that suggest other narratives. The AIDS quilt comes quickly to mind, as well as the emphasis on hospice and on emotional support for those infected with the virus.

There was a time when Christians prayed, with great sincerity, to be preserved from a sudden death. That prayer is still a part of the Book of Common Prayer. Nowadays, people might be more likely to pray *for* a sudden death. That tells us something: the story has changed. It also tells us that it can change again.

NURSING AS METAPHOR

CLAIRE FAGIN and DONNA DIERS are registered nurses who wrote this article while faculty members at the University of Pennsylvania and Yale University respectively. Published in New England Journal of Medicine *(1983), the article has be-*

come a classic. Fagin is currently president of the National League for Nursing.

For some time now we have been curious about the reactions of people we meet socially to being told, "I am a nurse." First reactions to this statement include the comment, "I never met a nurse socially before"; stories about the person's latest hospitalization, surgery, or childbearing experiences; the question "How can you bear handling bedpans [vomit, blood]?" or the remark, "I think I need another drink." We believe the statements reflect the fact that nursing evokes disturbing and discomforting images that many educated, middle-class, upwardly mobile Americans find difficult to handle in a social situation. As nurses, we are educated to give comfort, so it is something of a paradox when we make ourselves and others uncomfortable socially.

It is easy to say that some reactions are based on an underlying attitude toward nurses that we tend to think of as a stereotype. But labeling the attitude does not help us explain it or escape it. Perhaps we can deal with the social perception by examining the metaphors that underlie the concept of "nurse"—metaphors that influence not only language but also thought and action. An exploration of the metaphorical underpinnings of nursing must start with the etymology of the word "nurse," which is derived from the Latin for "nourish."

Nursing is a metaphor for mothering. Nursing has links with nurturing, caring, comforting, the laying on of hands, and other maternal types of behavior, all of which are seen in our society as essentially mundane and hardly worth noticing. Even the thought of the vertical nurse over the horizontal patient evokes regressed feelings in a woman or man who is told, "I am a nurse." Adults do not like to be reminded, especially in an adult, socially competitive setting, of the child who remains inside all of us.

Nursing is a metaphor for class struggle. Not only does nursing represent women's struggles for equality, but its position in the health world is that of the classic underdog, struggling to be heard, approved, and recognized. Nurses constitute the largest occupational group in the health-care system (1.6 million). They work predominantly in settings that are dominated by physicians and in which physicians represent the upper and controlling class. Dominant groups yield ground reluctantly, especially to those who are regarded as having simply settled for a job instead of choosing a more prestigious profession.

Nursing is a metaphor for equality. Little social distance separates the nurse from the patient or the patient from other patients in the nursing-care setting, no matter what the social class of each. Nurses themselves make little distinction in rank among persons with widely varying amounts of education. Nurses are perceived as members of the working class, and although this perception is valuable to the patient when he or she is ill and wants to be comforted, it may be awkward to encounter one's nurses at a black-tie reception, where working-class people do not belong.

Among physicians, nursing may be a metaphor for conscience. Nurses see all that happens in the name of health care—the neglect as well as the cures, the reasons for failure as well as those for success. The anxiety, not to mention the guilt, engendered by what nurses may know can be considerable. Nurses recognize that many of the physician's attempts to conquer death do not work. They are an uncomfortable reminder of fallibility.

Nursing is a metaphor for intimacy. Nurses are involved in the most private aspects of people's lives, and they cannot hide behind technology or a veil of omniscience as other practitioners or technicians in hospitals may do. Nurses do for others publicly what healthy persons do for themselves behind closed doors. Nurses, as trusted peers, are there to hear secrets, especially the ones born of vulnerability. Nurses are treasured when these interchanges are successful, but most often people do not wish to remember their vulnerability or loss of control, and nurses are indelibly identified with those terribly personal times.

Thanks to the worst of this kind of thinking, nursing is a metaphor for sex. Having seen and touched the bodies of strangers, nurses are perceived as willing and able sexual partners. Knowing and experienced, they unlike prostitutes, are thought, to be safe—a quality suggested by the cleanliness of their white uniforms and their professional aplomb.

Something like the sum of these images makes up the psychological milieu in which nurses live and work. Little wonder, then, that some of us have been badgered (at least in our earlier days) about our choice of career. Little wonder, then, that nurses have had to develop a resilience required of few other professionals. Little wonder, too, that it is so difficult for us to reply to our detractors. One may wonder why any self-respecting, reasonably intellectual man or woman chooses nursing as a lifelong career. Our students at Pennsylvania and Yale are regularly asked questions like this by family, friends, and acquaintances: "Why on earth are you becoming a nurse? You have the brains to be a (doctor, lawyer, other)." All of them, long before entering schools such as ours, must answer this question for themselves and their questioners in a way that permits them to begin and to continue nursing. Their responses and ours frequently focus on the role of the nurse, the variety and mobility possible in a nursing career, or the changing nature of the profession. That kind of answer doesn't get to the heart of the problem in the mind of the questioner. Although it may elicit an "Oh, I didn't realize that," it doesn't make any permanent points for anyone. The right answer has to address the metaphors, since these are the reasons for the concern. The answer must convey the feeling of satisfaction derived from the caring role; indifference to power for its own sake; the recognition that one is a doer who enjoys doing for and with others; but most of all, the pleasure associated with helping others from the position of a peer rather than from the assumed subordinate position of some other professions.

The metaphors, if we turn them around, can easily work to explain our position. Intimacy—why shrink from the word, even while we educate our listeners about its finer meaning—equality, conscience, and the many qualities of motherhood (another word that can usefully be separated from its stereotype) are exactly what draw people into nursing and keep them there.

If we could manage to be wistfully amused by the reactions we evoke at social events rather than defensive, life would be easier. Educated, middle-class, upwardly mobile—we are indeed the peers of others at these social gatherings. We are peers informed about disease prevention, the promotion of health, and rehabilitation. We are not disinterested experts but advocates, even for those who misinterpret us. Others may be only dimly aware of our role, but it is rooted deep in our history and exemplified by the great nursing leaders who have moved society forward: Lavinia Dock, so active in pursuing women's rights; Lillian Wald (a nurse whom society has preferred to disguise as a social worker), who developed the Henry Street Settlement and educated all of us in understanding and approaching health and social problems; Margaret Sanger, who faced disdain, ignominy, and imprisonment in her struggle to educate the public about birth control, and Sister Kenny, who was once the only hope for polio victims.

So much for the metaphors of others. For ourselves? We think of ourselves as Florence Nightingale—tough, canny, powerful, autonomous, and heroic.

> An important way of tracing nursing's heritage is through diaries and journals and biographies. A brief passage on historiography and self-profiles by nurses of very different times and circumstances appear here. However, our libraries contain many such selections and they could constitute an entire course in nursing literature.

WOMEN WORTHIES IN NURSING HISTORY

NANCY L. NOEL is Assistant Professor, Doctoral Program, Marion A. Buckley School of Nursing, Adelphi University, and has served as Curator of the Nursing Archives, Mugar Memorial Library, Boston University. She is recognized as a visible force in the resurgence of the nursing history movement. This selection appeared in the Western Journal of Nursing Research *in 1988.*

Biography as a form of historical inquiry has had a long past. The study of a life helps one understand a time, a person. It is a form of immortality, it can be a template, mirror, or example from which one can enhance one's own life. Biography can be scholarly research and lively entertainment. It is a literary genre with broad public appeal and as such can be a powerful tool in building institutions, reputations, and professions. Only a handful of nurses' biographies have been published. Women in general are woefully underrepresented in the biographical form. The worthy nurses who are subjects of biography have been mostly controversial figures whose lives touched broad segments of their cultures. They have been public figures, such as Margaret Sanger, Lillian Wald, and Emma Goldman. . . .

The person who chooses to study life needs a philosophy that values individualism and a firm commitment to truth. The biographer needs to be able to comprehend a subject developing through a life and immersed in a time. The biographer needs to understand a person's character as it is operationalized in career activities and range of influence. The right questions need to be asked about the meaning of a nurse's life. The scholar takes great responsibility in presenting that life to the public, choosing what invisibility may become visible.

The scholarly community and the lay public read biography. It helps transmit culture from one generation to the next. Let us encourage nurses to write biographies of our nurse women worthies. Let us document their efforts to improve health care and sanitation and to reduce infant and maternal mortality, thereby emancipating other women. These precursors for liberty, opportunity, and upward mobility have been central to American culture. Nurses as individuals and collectively have made significant contributions to improving health in this country. Their life stories are worthy of being told. (pp. 106–108)

THE CALL COMES

LYDIA HOLMAN went to the mountains of North Carolina on Christmas Day in 1900 to nurse an ill woman. Her story was first published in The Visiting Nurse Quarterly *in 1912. It was later reproduced in* Public Health Nursing *in 1937.*

All preparations to enjoy Christmas had been made, except reporting off duty—a most important thing for a nurse to do. On reaching the office, the act of reporting off was interrupted by the registrar's information. "A request has been received from some unknown place in the mountains for a nurse who can take all the responsibility of a typhoid fever case. The place is thirty miles from a railroad, regular physicians, or supplies of any kind, and is in a forest. You must go and take supplies."

Christmas day, early in the afternoon, the railway journey of twenty hours was over. At the little town station were a few people—the innkeeper, some travelers, and the liveryman, but no team. The difference of customs in different localities began to appear, and with them difficulties. The liveryman being asked for his best team, as ordered by telegram, remonstrates: "That place is thirty miles yon side of big mountain, the roads well-nigh impassable. No one, miners, lumbermen, or drummers are traveling over that mountain. No horses can get over these roads."

The innkeeper, liveryman, and the few travelers joined in estimating the journey out of the question until weather conditions should be better. It became quite evident to me that these men had never been taught the lesson of "getting there." I moralized, persuaded, demanded, and offered good pay for a team. Reach the sick woman that night I must. Two good horses, a heavy hack with the trunk well strapped to it, and a Negro driver at last were ready.

Ten hours to do eighteen miles from the base to the top of the mountain. As I ascended the clouds, the scenery became more wonderful, the air electrical, and biting cold; and the witchery of the clearest moonlight over tumbling streams, little waterfalls, deep precipices, high naked trees and beautiful underbrush tinged with frost, stimulated my mind, while my weary body rolled from side to side of the big wagon. Plowing through mud, ruts, over stumpy roads and river beds, the horses grew perceptibly weary, and the black driver sulky, as the miles grew slowly less.

One turn in the road looked over a high precipice into a moonlit field with deadened girdled trees. The shadows made weird outlines, and the driver crouched low in his seat. "Are you cold?" I asked.

"No mum."

"You're afraid. Why?"

"Well, them white things moving, they's ghosts." No amount of explanation could dispel the idea; the drummers had often told him so. He was full of fear, though the "ghosts" looked miles below. I asked for the whip, promising to keep all danger off. His only comment in handing the whip was, "You isn't afraid of anything."

At the top of the mountain at midnight, it took long and loud hallowing to awaken the proprietor of a cabin, where a stop of five hours was made. It was bewildering to be ushered into a room with a big fireplace full of blazing logs, the back log sizzling, the fire logs crackling, making light enough to see only beds and people. So few the beds, and so many heads peeping above the covers! . . .

About noon the next day I reached my patient. I found her desperately ill, receiving only the crude care of a good-hearted, though frightened mountain man. Soon I found myself installed as physician, nurse, housekeeper and maid-of-all work for two. Those were busy days, and nights too, spent for weeks at the patient's bedside.

In six weeks the patient was out, going about the place, making a great impression on the mountain folk. Typhoid with them is fatal, and the most dreaded of diseases. Their curiosity and interest were thoroughly aroused, so they came to the patient's home, complaining of every conceivable ill. . . .

This was the beginning of 37 years in the mountains. (pp. 702–703)

KÓPASKER, ICELAND

REGINA STEFNISDÓTTIR, a nurse from Iceland, wrote this personal account of her work in an isolated village as a special offering to On Nursing *and you, its readers.*

Kópasker is a long way from Perth, Western Australia. This I say because I happened to work in hospitals in Perth during 1969–1971 and I felt the South Pole at my doorstep. During 1976–1978 I was a district nurse in Kópasker in the northeast of Iceland. Then I had the feeling of living on top of the world, under the shadow of the North Pole. For some, the jump between these two places is a big one. For me it was to pack two suitcases and go ahead. Now, no doctor was available, so a nurse had to be the next best choice.

We moved to Kópasker the 15th of August 1976: my husband, our black spitz sledgedog and me. I had never laid my eyes on this isolated place and knew next to nothing about it. Minimum housing expenses were supposed to be a part of the bargain. We discovered that the house was a two floor mansion called Umsvalir and had been built in the forties shortly after the second world war for the district doctor to live in. We were supposed to live on the upper floor and the health station was downstairs. Four doctors from Husavik hospital came alternately every Tuesday afternoon and stayed for three hours.

Snow is often extremely heavy in these parts and sometimes sets in very early in autumn. The area may be expected to be closed off for longer or shorter periods of time during midwinter. It meant that it would be difficult to keep in contact with the nearest town of Husavik let alone Akureyri where there is a rather big hospital. At this time I was 41 years old and had an unusual background in nursing. I had been nurse director in a little hospital on the east coast, a nurse in pediatrics in Algeria, a general duties nurse in a casualty clinic in Reykjavik, a visiting nurse in the Reykjavik City Health Center attending babies and infants and doing different duties in rehabilitation nursing in Perth and Sydney, Australia. I had worked in a polyclinic in Texas, USA, on a medical-surgical floor and later worked in a blood bank in Reykjavik collecting blood and doing some research work. I tell you this because the experience turned out to be a big asset when I became a nurse in such a remote area.

A wave of warmth strikes me when I think back to Kópasker. I don't know why. Since then I've been many places. Probably it is because this small community needed me and the responsibility was mine alone.

When I arrived, the very first thing that came to my mind was: How in the world am I to supervise this unit as well as possible under these circumstances? A map of the area was a must, and I drew a circle around "my piece." The next thing was to learn by heart all the farms, big or small, and their situation; that is, whether they were situated near the sea, or inland. Next I called the national citizen registry and asked them for a list of names, ages, and addresses for each and every one who was a permanent resident in the area. Inhabitants numbered around 340 at that time in Kópasker village and the sheep farms nearby. I tried to be quick in memorizing the farms and whether they were extremely isolated; names and ages of their residents, who was young and who was old? By doing this I felt I could prepare myself better for what to expect. Later I was told that the saying went amongst people: "This nurse is pretty peculiar. How come she knows us all?"

Then the typical stress periods came. A boys' summer camp was opened early in summer, around the middle of June until the middle of September. About sixty lively boys ages 6 to 12 were added to the crowd and of course the people who attended them. No health personnel, mind you. A flood of summer tourists came and also visitors staying in summer cottages.

Came September and October and sheep were collected from summer pastures to be slaughtered to store up meat before winter. Then a large group of guest workers worked at the slaughterhouse. No addition to the health personnel, of course.

Today, when I think back, I feel that something new and exciting happened every day. I repaired a cat's hind leg, sutured an eyelid on a fine riding horse, a twenty centimeter suture on a breast of a favorite riding horse who belonged to one of the ladies on a farm. One day I opened the door to the waiting room and said: Next please! Then I heard: "Meeeee." A newborn lamb had broken a leg so the easiest way of all was to bring it to the health station. The veterinarian was a good two hours' drive away.

The chores did not lack variety. Immunity shots for groups, if influenza was expected, preparing for the eye doctor on his yearly visits, receiving the team who visited for cancer screening, attending the pharmacy all around the clock, teaching the kids sex education. That was the only teaching I was asked for. Ordinary teachers covered the rest of the health education curriculum. I dragged a boy from underneath a farming machine and travelled long distances for sick patient visits. Drove people to airplanes when leaving for the hospital to Akureyri or Reykjavik. Sutured wounds a lot, removed a few nails from fingers, and pressed dentin into teeth. I could go on forever. Of course, not to forget my doctor who came every Tuesday afternoon. So I collected patients during the week and organized his three hours' stay.

The salary was meager but I forgot about the value of money. Fresh fish was on my doorstep many a morning. Someone had gone fishing in the early hours and remembered me. A bag of mushrooms, meat or potatoes somebody had sneaked through the door to pay me for some little thing I'd done for them. It was wonderful.

One little incident is clearer than anything in my memory; the telephone rang one fine day the second summer of my stay. I was told that a two-month-old filly had run into a barbed wire fence and injured herself badly. This was a premium horse to be. I called the vet and got his permission to attend the animal if I could manage. He himself was extremely busy and said that the best thing would probably be to shoot the little one. I collected the necessary things and tools I imagined I would need and drove off. When I arrived at the site, a big herd of horses was gathered in one corner of a fenced pasture. The filly lay scared stiff in her blood. I observed the laceration and discovered a 10–15 centimeter long, deep cut inside the upper part of the right front leg. Three men were there from the farm to assist and they drove off the other horses. I cuddled the little one for a while trying to build up some trust between us. I talked to her and tried to comfort her as I could and let her smell my body as she pleased. Then I gave anesthesia and waited some and started sewing. The little animal lay dead still. I concentrated on what I was doing and did not notice anything else. I was apprehensive; happenings like this one were not my daily cup of coffee. All of a sudden I sensed an extra force into my being. I looked up and met the eyes of the mare, the mother horse. We looked each other in the eye for a moment. She stood there, every nerve and muscle tense to the full, watching every move of mine, ready to strike if something happened she did not like. Never in the twenty-something years I'd worked in nursing had I experienced anything like this. It was like we talked to each other without words. She said: "I notice exactly what you are doing." I felt like saying: "I'm trying the very best I can." She said: "I can see that." This happened in a break of a second and filled me with confidence. She stood there, proud and erect, watching, until everything was over. Then she came nearer, rubbed herself into her youngster, and they walked away slowly. The farmer removed the stitches on time and said it was unnecessary to call me because everything had turned out so well. My role, of course, was over this time.

People who are in close contact with animals experience this all the time, I presume. I have not read about it, or else may not have noticed. For me this was a unique experience.

When you finish reading this you may think that nursing animals was my main duty up there. On the contrary. I tried to do what was needed and expected of me. Everything was one: man, animals, the land and the sea. I had the privilege of being a participant and I enjoyed every moment.

Lady Luck was with me; nobody died while I was there.

After those wonderful two years I said goodbye with mixed feelings. When I was leaving somebody said: "Why don't you go to Thorshoefn (a village a little bigger further east); there is a doctor over there." My snappy answer was: "No thanks, I know who goes on fishing trips and who minds the store."

> It could be said that, in many ways, the act of nursing is in itself poetry in motion. Nursing, like poetry, has its own rhythms, its own beauty, its own evocative power. However, nurses often directly express themselves through the act of writing poetry, and such selections have been seeded throughout this book. Included here are four segments by poets about poetry.

I Dream a World

Margaret Walker Alexander published her first book of poetry, For My People, *in 1942 and the historical novel* Jubilee *in 1966. Her poem, "For My People," has become one of the literary*

anthems of the Black community. Her biography, Richard
Wright: Daemonic Genius, *was published in 1988. After four
decades of teaching, she retired as Emeritus Professor of English
at Jackson State University in Jackson, Mississippi.*

My mother read poetry to me before I could read, and I can't remember when I couldn't read. We grew up with books. I don't
think you can write if you don't read. You can't read if you can't
think. Thinking, reading, and writing all go together. When I was
about eight, I decided that the most wonderful thing, next to a human being, was a book.

I finished grade school when I was eleven and a half. I finished
high school when I was fourteen. I went to college when I was fifteen. I would have finished at eighteen but I had to stay out a
year. My father said I was precocious.

He told me the first three lessons I learned about poetry: you
must have pictures, you must have music, and you must have
meaning. And I learned that prose has to have rhythm, pictures,
and meaning, too.

I was twenty-two when I wrote "For My People." With the exception of the last stanza, I wrote it in fifteen minutes on a typewriter. That was one of those things that came out whole. That's
been more than fifty years ago and I haven't changed in my idea.
I've read that poem all over the country . . . .

I taught nearly forty years and I taught my students that every
person is a human being. Every human personality is sacred, potentially divine. Nobody is any more than that and nobody can be
any less. (p. 115)

POETRY IS . . .

*ROSARIO MORALES is a Puerto Rican American feminist, mother of
three, student of science and anthropology, who broke a lifetime
of silence to write for* This Bridge Called My Back *(1983). This
selection is from* Getting Home Alive *(1986).*

> Poetry is
> something refined in your vocabulary
> taking its place at the table in a

silver bowl:
essence of culture. (p. 40)

SISTER/OUTSIDER

AUDRE LORDE (1934–1992) described herself as a Black woman warrior poet; she was also a teacher, a political activist, and a mother. She wrote many books, including two on her 14-year battle with breast cancer: The Cancer Journals *and* A Burst of Light.

The distillation from which true poetry springs births thought as dream births concept, as feeling births idea, as knowledge births (precedes) understanding. . . .

For women, then, poetry . . . is a vital necessity of our existence. It forms the quality of light within which we predicate our hopes and dreams toward survival and change, first made into language, then into idea, then into more tangible action. Poetry is the way we help give name to the nameless so it can be thought. The farthest horizons of our hopes and fears are cobbled by our poems carved from the rock experiences of our daily lives. (p. 37)

EDUCATION BY POETRY

ROBERT FROST first presented Education by Poetry: A Meditative Monologue *as a talk to the Amherst College Alumni Council in 1930. It was later included in* Selected Prose of Robert Frost.

I want to add one thing more that the experience of poetry is to anyone who comes close to poetry. There are two ways of coming close to poetry. One is by writing poetry. And some people think I want people to write poetry, but I don't; that is, I don't necessarily. I only want people to write poetry if they want to write poetry. I have never encouraged anybody to write poetry that did not want to write it, and I have not always encouraged those who did want to write it. That ought to be one's own funeral. It is a hard, hard life, as they say.

. . . there is another way to come close to poetry, fortunately, and that is in the reading of it, not as linguistics, not as history, not as anything but poetry. . . .

The person who gets close enough to poetry, he is going to know more about the word *belief* than anybody else knows, even in religion nowadays.

. . . there is a literary belief. Every time a poem is written, every time a short story is written, it is written not by cunning, but by belief. The beauty, the something, the little charm of the thing to be, is more felt than known. . . . No one who has ever come close to the arts has failed to see the difference between things written . . . with cunning and device, and the kind that are believed into existence, that begin in something more felt than known. This you can realize quite as well—not quite as well, perhaps, but nearly as well—in reading as you can in writing. I would undertake to separate short stories on that principle; stories that have been believed into existence and stories that have been cunningly devised. And I could separate the poems still more easily.

*   *   *

This chapter, as promised, has only touched upon the questions: Why should nurses write? And how and what could we add to the literature, as we have sampled and savored its beauty and power throughout this volume? Our literary celebration ends on a personal note.

What tales do *you* have to tell? What thoughts do *you* have to share? What literary form best captures and conveys *your* intent? The essay, narrative, poem, journal, editorial?

Yes, writing is an act of courage, as well as an act of commitment, conviction, and confidence. It requires self-discipline; it involves exposing our ideas to public scrutiny and thereby risking rejection. Yet, for all of the reasons mentioned in this chapter, writing is both a natural and essential act for nurses. For *you.*

As we turn this final page together, the last words are ours. Only we can say—and say well—that which we know best.

Note

1. JAMA, 11/3/89.

BIBLIOGRAPHY

Achterberg, J. (1990). *Woman as healer* (pp. 3–5, 190–191, 193–194). Boston: Shambhala Publications.

Alcott, L. M. (1984). *Hospital sketches* (1863) (pp. 47–64, 92–93). New York: Garland Publishing.

Alexander, M. W. (1989). In B. Lanker (Ed.), *I dream a world* (p. 115). New York: Stewart, Tabori & Chang, Inc.

Allende, I. (1989). Interminable life. *The stories of Eva Luna* (pp. 261–275). New York: Atheneum.

Angelou, M. (1989). Introduction. In B. Lanker (Ed.), *I dream a world*. New York: Stewart, Tabori & Chang, Inc.

Anonymous (1988). Hello David, my name is Dusty. *California Nursing Review, 10*(5), cover.

Anzaldúa, G. (1983). Foreword: What to do from here and how? In C. Moraga & G. Anzaldúa (Eds.), *This bridge called my back* (pp. iv–v). Latham, NY: Kitchen Table.

Aptheker, B. (1989). *Tapestries of life: Women's work, women's consciousness* (pp. 39–41), 253–254). Amherst, MA: The University of Massachusetts Press.

Armstrong, D. (1992). If you can walk, you can dance. In *CGFNS President's report, ANA House of Delegates, July, 1992*. New York: American Journal of Nursing Company.

Armstrong, P., & Feldman, S. (1986). *A midwife's story*. New York: Arbor House.

Baer, E. D. (1993). *A generous death*. Unpublished essay.

Bateson, M. C. (1990). *Composing a life* (pp. 142–146, 156–161, 239–241). New York: Plume (Penguin).

Beethoven, L. V. (1802/1961). In E. Anderson (Ed.), Heiligenstadt testament, *The Letters of Beethoven* (October 6, 1802). Reprinted in *Health* May/June, 1989, 90 with permission from W. W. Norton.

Bellah, R., Madsen, R., Sullivan, W. M., Swiddler, A., & Tipton, S. M. (1985). *Habits of the heart* (p. 194). New York: Harper & Row.

Bevis, E. O., & Watson, J. (1989). *Toward a caring curriculum: A new pedagogy for nursing*. New York: National League for Nursing.

Billingsley, M. (1990). The Saudi experience. *Nursing Connections, 3*(4), 19.

Bird, R. (1992, Winter). A daughter's story. *Stanford Nurse*, pp. 12–13.

Black, B. P. (1992). *Caring in hellish places*. Unpublished essay.

Buchanan, J. H. (1985, November/December). Patient encounters: The experience of disease. Charlottesville, VA: University Press of Virginia, pp. 70–77, 82–86, 141–143.

Buddha. We are what we think.

Butler, S. (1903). *The way of all flesh*.

Califano, J. A. (1992). The nurse as a revolutionary. *The Academic Nurse: Journal of the School of Nursing of Columbia University, 10*(1), 14–19.

Callahan, D. (1990). The priority of care over cure. In *What kind of life* (pp. 143–145, 149). New York: Simon & Schuster.

Carter, L. (1991, July). Only human. *Western Journal of Medicine,* p. 82.

Castañeda, L. (1986). Cashier & line stocker. In M. R. Michelson & M. R. Dressler (Eds.), *Women and Work: Photographs and personal writings* (p. 78). Troutdale, OR: NewSage Press.

Chao, Y-M. (1992). A unique concept of nursing care. *International Nursing Review, 39*(6), 181.

Chen, Y-C (1988). You and I. *A Taoist model for human caring: The lived experiences and caring needs of mothers with children suffering from cancer in Taiwan.* Doctoral dissertation.

Chinn, P. L. (1989, February). Nursing patterns of knowing and feminist thought. *Nursing & Health Care, 10*(2), pp. 71–75.

Christ, C. (1980). *Diving deep and surfacing: Women writers on spiritual quest* (p. 1). Boston: Beacon Press.

Cliff, M. (1980). Claiming an identity they taught me to despise (pp. 41–42). Watertown, MA: Persephone Press.

Clifton, L. (1976). Generations. *Generations: A memoir* (p. 78). New York: Random House.

Collins, B. T. (1988, November/December). Letter to the editor. *California Nursing Review.*

Collins, J. (1986). Midwives. In M. R. Michelson & M. R. Dressler (Eds.), *Women and work: Photographs and personal writings* (p. 147). Troutdale, OR: NewSage Press.

Cousins, N. (1979). *Anatomy of an illness as perceived by the patient: Reflections on healing and regeneration* (pp. 67–69, 72–74, 133, 153–154). New York: W. W. Norton.

Cousins, N. (1983). *The healing heart: Antidotes to panic and helplessness* (pp. 15–16, 112–113, 229–232). New York: W. W. Norton.

Cousins, N. (1982). Writers and physicians: Toward a common culture. *Archives of Internal Medicine, 142,* pp. 2160–2162. [Not a direct quote; a reference in text only]

Cowan, J. (1992). Mother's day. *Small decencies: Reflections and meditations on being human at work* (pp. 99–101). New York: Harper Business.

Cowan, J. (1992). The sailing instructor. *Small decencies: Reflections and meditations on being human at work* (p. 117). New York: Harper Business.

Curtin, L. (1990). Maria's choice. *Nursing Management, 21*(11), 7–8.

Dass, R., & Gorman, P. (1990). *How can I help?* (pp. 28–28, 54–55, 58, 62–64, 67–69). New York: Random House.

de Beauvoir, S. (1965). *A very easy death* [tr. Patrick O'Brien]. New York: Random House.

Deborah, Genesis 35, Verses 6–8, *The Bible.*

Dickinson, E. (1955). Hope is a thing with feathers. In T. H. Johnson (Ed.), *The poems of Emily Dickinson* (p. 30). Cambridge, MA: The Belknap Press of Harvard University Press.

Dickinson, E. (1982). The mystery of pain. In *Collected poems* (p. 10). New York: Avenel Books.

Dickinson, E. (1955). There's been a death. In T. H. Johnson (Ed.), *The poems of Emily Dickinson.* Cambridge, MA: The Belknap Press of Harvard University Press.

Diers, D. (1991). Learning: The art and craft of nursing. *American Journal of Nursing, 91*(1), 65–66.

Dock, L. L. (1900). The nurses' settlement in New York. *Short papers on nursing subjects* (pp. 27–35). Published by M. Louise Longeway. Reprinted by Garland Publishing.

Doctorow, E. L. (1991). Planning to write . . . In J. Charlton (Ed.), *The writer's quotation book* (3rd rev.). Wainscott, NY: Pushcart Press.

Donahue, M. P. (1991). The spirit of nursing. *Journal of Professional Nursing, 7*(3), 149.

Donahue, M. P. (1991). Why nursing history? *Journal of Professional Nursing, 7*(2), 77.

Donne, J. (1977). Death be not proud. In A. J. Smith (Ed.), *The complete English poems*. New York: Penguin Books.

Eliot, T. S. (1962). The love song of J. Alfred Prufrock. In *The complete poems and plays*. Philadelphia: Harcourt Brace Jovanovich.

Estes, C. P. (1992). *Women who run with the wolves: Myths and stories of the wild woman archetype* (p. 463). New York: Ballantine.

Eyjolfsdottir, S. (1989). [Poems III and IX]. *Elegy to my son*. Reykjavik, Iceland: BOKRUN Ltd.

Fagin, C., & Diers, D. (1983). Nursing as metaphor. *New England Journal of Medicine, 309*, pp. 116–117.

Feuerstein, M-T. (1991). *Why is it difficult to sell maternal mortality?* Unpublished poem.

Fishbein, J. (1990). The poetry of medicine. *Journal of the American Medical Association, 264*(23), 2999.

Francis, P. (1975). The autumn of my life. *Congressional Record*, April 22, 1975.

Frank, A. W. (1991). *At the will of the body* (pp. 55–58, 68–71, 129–135). Boston: Houghton Mifflin.

Freund, C. (1990). *The unity of education, research and practice: A kaleidoscopic view of nursing* (pp. 20–24). Kansas City, MO: American Nurses Association.

Frost, R. (1966). Education by poetry: A meditative monologue. In H. Cox & E. C. Lathem (Eds.), *Selected prose*. New York: Holt, Rinehart & Winston.

Frost, R. (1979). The road not taken. In E. C. Lathem (Ed.), *The poetry of Robert Frost* (p. 105). New York: Henry Holt and Company.

Fuentes, C. (1992). Quoted in G. Garcia, Daring dreamer, *Time*, June 29, 1992, p. 78.

Goodrich, A. W. (1932). The nurses and ethics. In *The social and ethical significance of nursing* (p. 14). New York: Macmillan.

Gordon, S. (1992, September/October). What nurses know. *Mother Jones*, pp. 41–46.

Gordon, S. (1991). *Prisoners of men's dreams: Striking out for a new feminine future* (pp. 145, 154). Boston: Little, Brown.

Grant-Mackie, D. (1992). *Koroua*. Unpublished poem. Submitted by author.

Hall, S. (1990, November-December). Gail. *Health*, pp. 62–69.

Hammarskjöld, D. (1941, 1966). *Markings* (Leif Sjöberg & W. H. Auden, trans.). New York: Alfred A. Knopf and Faber & Faber Ltd.

Hansen, C. B. (1975). The gift. *Balancing act: A book of poems by Maine women*. Portland, ME: Littoral Books.

Havel, V. (1989). *Letters of Olga* (p. 237). New York: First Owl Book Edition.

Hedgeman, A. A. (1989). Anna Arnold Hedgeman. In B. Lanker (Ed.), *I dream a world* (p. 90). New York: Stewart, Tabori & Chang, Inc.

Hegevary, S. (1991). Something to believe in. *Journal of Professional Nursing, 7*(2), 76.

Henderson, V. (1971, March). Health is everybody's business. *The Canadian Nurse*, pp. 32–34.

Holman, L. (1937). Two Christmas stories. *Public Health Nursing, 29*(12), 702–703.

Joseph, J. (1991). Warning. In S. Martz (Ed.), *When I am an old woman I shall wear purple*. Watsonville, CA: Papier Mache Press.

Keller, H. (1957). *The Open Door*.

King, M. L. (1963). *I have a dream.* Speech delivered at the Lincoln Memorial, Washington, DC, August 28, 1963.

King, M. L. (1968). *Trumpet of conscience.* New York: Harper & Row.

Koller, A. (1990). Working. *The stations of solitude* (pp. 41–42). New York: William Morrow.

Kroener, J. (1992). Letter to editors of *On nursing: A literary celebration,* citing Helen Keller, "There are red letter days."

Lenburg, C. (1988). Out of the hard places. In T. Schorr & A. Zimmerman (Eds.), *Making choices, taking chances: Nurse leaders tell their stories* (p. 205). St. Louis: C. V. Mosby.

Lerner, M. (1990). *Wrestling with the angel: A memoir of my triumph over illness* (pp. 48–52, 90–94, 109–110). New York: W. W. Norton.

Lessard, S. (1980). Talk of the town. *The New Yorker,* August 11, 22.

Lester, C. (1975). Carmelita Lester. In S. Terkel (Ed.), *Working* (pp. 650–655). New York: Avon Books.

LeSueur, M. (1982). Rites of ancient ripening. In *Ripening: Selected works, 1927–1980.* New York: The Feminist Press at The City University of New York.

Levino, S. (1989). The healing for which we took birth. In R. Carlson & B. Shield (Eds.), *Healers on Healing* (pp. 196–199). Los Angeles: Jeremy P. Tarcher Inc.

Lindbergh, A. M. (1956). Broken Shell. *The unicorn and other poems: 1935–1955* (p. 82). New York: Random House.

Lindbergh, A. M. (1956). Family album. *The unicorn and other poems: 1935–1955* (pp. 79–81). New York: Random House.

Linfield, D. (1991). How do I tell my daughter? *New York Times,* June 3, 1992.

Livingston, G. (1992). Dear Lucas. In the San Francisco Chronicle, *Image Magazine,* November 8, pp. 28–29.

Longfellow, H. W. (1886). Santa Filomena. *Longfellow's poems* (p. 222). Cambridge: The Riverside Press.

Lorde, A. (1984). *Sister/outsider: Essays & speeches* (p. 37). Trumansburg, NY: The Crossing Press.

Machiavelli, N. *The prince.*

Mallison, M. (1987). How can you bear to be a nurse? *American Journal of Nursing, 87*(5), 419.

Masson, V. (1991). The art of the matter. *Nursing Outlook, 39*(4), 187.

Mennis, B. (1977). Gardens, growth and community. *Women: A Journal of Liberation, 5*(2), 44.

Millay, E. S. V. (1956). To the wife of a sick friend. In N. Millay (Ed.), *Collected poems* (pp. 209–210). New York: Harper & Row.

Millay, E. S. V. (1956). Lament. In N. Millay (Ed.), *Collected poems* (pp. 103–104). New York: Harper & Row.

Miller, E. E. (1989). Trust and honesty: Foundations of healing. In R. Carlson & B. Shield (Eds.), *Healers on Healing* (p. 110). Los Angeles: Jeremy P. Tarcher Inc.

Milton, J. *On his blindness.*

Moccia, P. (1988). *Curriculum revolution: Agenda for change* (p. 63). New York: National League for Nursing.

Morales, A. L. (1983). And even Fidel can't change that. In C. Moraga & G. Anzaldúa (Eds.), *This bridge called my back.* Latham, NY: Kitchen Table.

Morales, R. (1986). *Getting home alive.* Ithaca, NY: Firebrand Books.

Morgan, R. (1990). Network of the imaginary mother. In *Upstairs in the garden.* Reprinted in G. Steinem (1992). Bodies of knowledge. *Revolution from within: A book of self-esteem* (p. 248). New York: Little, Brown.

Morgan, R. (1989). The two Gretels. In J. Canan (Ed.), *She rises like the sun.* Freedom, CA: The Crossing Press.

Niemira, D. A. (1982). A time to decide. *Journal of the American Medical Association, 267*(14), 1913.

Nightingale, F. (1990). Ever yours (Let us be anxious). In Vicinus, M., & Nergaard, B. (Eds.), *Florence Nightingale: Selected letters* (p. 386). Cambridge, MA: Harvard University Press.

Nightingale, F. (1872). For us who nurse.

Nightingale, F. (1856–57). I stand at the altar (Private note).

Nightingale, F. (1856, August). If I could only (Private note).

Nightingale, F. (1959). It is often thought. In *Notes on nursing: What it is and what it is not.* In Duckworth edition.

Nightingale, F. (1866, September 13). Letter to Dr. William Farr.

Nightingale, F. (1857, February). No one can feel for the Army as I do. (Private note).

Nightingale, F. (1867, April). Nursing is an art. To the Editor, *Macmillan's Magazine.*

Nightingale, F. (1854, January). Our vocation is a difficult one. Letter to her cousin Marianne.

Nightingale, F. When I entered into service. In E. Huxley (Ed.), *Florence Nightingale* (p. 53). New York: Putnam's & Sons.

Noel, N. L. (1988). Historiography: Biography or "women worthies" in nursing history. *Western Journal of Nursing Research, 10*(1), 106–108.

Noonan, D. (1989). *Neuro: Life on the frontlines of brain surgery and neurological medicine* (pp. 11–13, 158–159, 218–219). New York: Simon and Schuster.

Novello, J. N. (1984). Only as high as I can reach. *1986 annual report, Pennsylvania State Board of Nurse Examiners.*

Odenbach, G. (1990). *An Anasazi woman speaks.* (pp. 1–2). Watsonville, CA: Papier Mache Press.

Olds, S. (1989). The line. In *The dead and the living* (p. 54). New York: Alfred A. Knopf.

Olsen, T. (1961). I stand here ironing. In *Tell me a riddle* (p. 75). Philadelphia: Lippincott.

Orwell, G. (1991). Writing a book . . . In J. Charlton (Ed.), *The writer's quotation book* (3rd rev.). Wainscott, NY: Pushcart Press.

Ozick, C. (1983). *New York Times.*

Parker, D. (1926/1954). The veteran. In *The portable Dorothy Parker.* New York: Viking Penguin.

Paterson, J. G., & Zderad, L. T. (1988). *Humanistic nursing* (p. 87). New York: National League for Nursing.

Pirtle, C. (1969). I'm not sad. In R. Lewis (Ed.), *Journeys: Prose by children of the English-speaking world* (p. 157). New York: Simon & Schuster.

Rich, A. (1978). Introduction (p. 7). In S. Miles et al. (Eds.), *Ordinary women/mujeres comunes.* New York: Ordinary Women.

Rich, A. (1976). *Of woman born: Motherhood as experience and institution* (p. 246). New York: W. W. Norton.

Roberts, M. (1980). Martha and Mary raise consciousness from the dead. In Z. Fairbairns et al. (Eds.), *Tales I tell my mother* (p. 72). Boston: South End Press.

Ross, J. (1989). *Fighting the enemy and other final chapters: Paying the price of our stories.* Unpublished presentation made at the West Coast Hastings Center 20th Anniversary Celebration, San Francisco.

Rowbotham, S. (1973). *Woman's Consciousness, Man's World* (p. 29). Middlesex: Penguin Books.

Rukeyser, M. (1976). Recovering. *The gates* (pp. 57–58). New York: McGraw Hill.

Sachs, G. A. (1988). On deeper reflection. *Journal of the American Medical Association, 259*(14), 2145.

Scarlett, E. P. (1991). Earle P. Scarlett (pp. 119–120). In R. Reynolds & J. Stone (Eds.), *On doctoring.* Princeton, NJ: Robert Wood Johnson Foundation.

Schweitzer, A. (1966). *Out of my life and thought: An autobiography* (pp. 240–243). (C. T. Campion, trans.) New York: Henry Holt.

Sexton, A. (1975). Courage. In *The awful rowing toward God* (pp. 425–426). Boston: Houghton Mifflin.

Sexton, A. (1981). Words. *The complete poems—Anne Sexton* (pp. 463–464). Boston: Houghton Mifflin.

Sharp, E. (1992, January). Down but not out (patient's advocate). *RN Magazine,* pp. 27–28.

Shaw, G. B. (1921). *Back to Methuselah,* Part I, Act I.

Sievers, M. K. (1989). Flashbacks: The character of pain. *American Journal of Nursing, 89*(5), 784.

Sleet, J. (1901). A successful experiment. *American Journal of Nursing, 1,* 729–731.

Snow, C. P. (1973). Human care. *Journal of the American Medical Association, 225*(6), 617–19.

Sontag, S. (1978). *Illness as metaphor* (p. 3). New York: Farrar, Straus and Giroux.

Stefnisdóttir, R. (1992). *Kópasker, Iceland.* Unpublished essay.

Steinem, G. (1992). Bodies of knowledge. *Revolution from within: A book of self-esteem* (pp. 244–248). New York: Little, Brown.

Stevens, W. (1965). The house was quiet and the world was calm. *The collected poems of Wallace Stevens.* New York: Alfred A. Knopf.

Stevenson, R. L. (1961). To Alison Cunningham (from her boy). *A child's garden of verses.* New York: Platt & Munk.

Stevenson, R. L. (1961). The land of counterpane. *A child's garden of verses.* New York: Platt & Munk.

Stilwell-Smith, J. *The legend of Edith Cavell, British nurse.*

Stone, J. (1980). Death. *In all this rain.* Baton Rouge, LA: Louisiana State University Press.

Stone, J. (1990). *In the country of hearts: Journeys in the art of medicine* (pp. 59–64, 67–71). New York: Delacorte Press.

Stoneman, D. (1986, January). The other side of Alzheimer's. *Present Time.* Reprinted in *Health* May/June, 1992, 86, 88–89.

Styles, M. (1992). Nightingale: The enduring symbol. *Notes on nursing* (pp. 72–75). Philadelphia: J.B. Lippincott Company.

The Mother. *Seeds of light.*

Tennyson, A. *The princess.*

Thomas, D. (1952). Do not go gentle into that good night. *Poems of Dylan Thomas* (p. 215). New York: New Directions Publishing Corp.

Thomas, L. (1983). Nurses. *The youngest science: Notes of a medicine watcher* (pp. 61–67). New York: Viking Press.

Thucydides. *The history of the Peloponnesian War.*

Tisdale, S. (1986). *The sorcerer's apprentice* (pp. 129–130). New York: McGraw Hill.

Truitt, A. (1982). *Daybook: The journal of an artist* (pp. 65–66, 171–175, 186–192). New York: Penguin, Pantheon Books.

Ufema, J. K. (1988). In T. Schorr & A. Zimmerman (Eds.), *Making choices, taking chances: Nurse leaders tell their stories* (pp. 360–361). St. Louis: C.V. Mosby.

UNICEF (1991). Facts for life: Women's work. New York: Author.

Wachter, R. M. (1991). The parable (on heaven and hell). *The fragile coalition: Scientists, activists, and AIDS.* New York: St. Martin's Press.

Walsh, L. V. (1990). The essence of midwifery. *Journal of Nurse Midwifery.*

Warren, R. P. (1978). Truth. In *Being Here: Poetry 1977–1980* (p. 63). New York: Random House.

Welty, E. (1984). *One writer's beginnings* (p. 10). Cambridge, MA: Harvard University Press.

Wolfe, T. (1940). *You can't go home, again.* New York: Harper & Row.

Wong, N. (1983). In search of the self as hero: Confetti of voices of New Year's night. In C. Moraga & G. Anzaldúa (Eds.), *This bridge called my back* (pp. 180–181). Latham, NY: Kitchen Table.

Woolf, V. (1938/1960). *Three guineas* (pp. 62–63). Philadelphia: Harcourt Brace Jovanovich.

Yamano, H. B. (1989). My mother's stories. In B. Aptheker, *Tapestries of life: Women's work, women's consciousness* (pp. 31–32). Amherst, MA: The University of Massachusetts Press.

Yorker, B. C. (1991). The rain and their dreams. *Journal of Child and Adolescent Psychopharmacology, 1*(4), 4.

CONTRIBUTORS

Listed below are the names of those who responded to our request to assist in identifying literature meaningful to nurses. We are most appreciative of their participation in this project. We regret that there was not space in this volume to include all of their suggestions, and we apologize if any persons were inadvertently omitted.

Respondents were from all part of the world. Mostly they answered for themselves alone, but some represented their national nurses associations in making suggestions.

Sarah Abrams
Clara Adams-Ender
Yang-Heui Ahn
Linda Aiken
Nisab Akhtar
Wayne Antoine
Doris Armstrong
Lauren Arnold
Ellen Baer
Judith Baigis-Smith
Patricia Benner
Molly Billingsley
Barbara Bishop
Beth Perry Black
Judith Black-Feather
Doris Bloch
Lisa Bonadonna
Fay Bower
Dagmar Brodt
Billye Brown
Mary Pierce Brosmer
Yu-Mei Chao
Rita Chow

Paula Christensen
June Clark
Trevor Clay
Mary Carolyn Cooper
Laurel Archer Copp
Inge Corless
Leah Curtin
Grace Davidson
Anne Davis
Bertha Davis
Vivien DeBack
Donna Diers
Mary Donaldson
Kathleen Dracup
Maurice Drake
Susan Dudas
Helen Dulock
Rhetaugh Dumas
Doris England
Linda Ennis
Glenora Erb
Helen Erickson
Claire Fagin

Veronica Feeg
Vernice Ferguson
Betty Ferrell
Juanita Fleming
Patricia Forni
Maryann Fralic
Betsy Frank
Marilyn Frank-Stromborg
Rita A. Frantz
Ellen French
Carol Germain
Carol Gold
Janet Gottschalk
Marcia Grant
Diana Grant-Mackie
Jim Grout
Ingibjorg Gunnarsdottir
Edward Halloran
Persis Mary Hamilton
Charlene Hanson
Andrea Harris
Marilyn Harris
Lulu Hassenplug

Joellen Hawkins
Jane Healey
Ann Henrick
Ada Sue Hinshaw
Jacqueline Hott
Kate Husk
Charlotte Isler
Susan Jacobsen
Marjorie Jamieson
Hazel Johnson-Brown
Karlene Kerfoot
Diane Kjervik
Mo-Im Kim
JoEllen Koerner
Dixie Koldjeski
Barbara Kozier
Janelle Krueger
Alice Kuramoto
Bernardine Lacey
Eleanor Lambertsen
Crystal Lange
Patricia Larson
Carrie Lenburg
Nan Leslie
Myra Levine
Iris L'Heritier
Sherlyn Loubert
Ruth Watson Lubic
Sally Lusk
Lois Malasanos
Beverly Malone
Joann Mapp
Ida Martinson
Veneta Masson
Barbara McArthur
Rosemary McCarthy
Joanne McCloskey
Margaret McClure
Beverly McElmurry

Gertrude Kay
    McFarland
Judith McFarlane
Deborah McGuire
Durga Mehta
Pamela Minarik
Zina Mirsky
Betty Mitsunaga
Lillian Mood
Randi Mortensen
Ildaura Murillo-Rohde
Narender Nagpal
Susan Neidlinger
Gwen Nissell
Marie Nolan
Elizabeth Norman
Mary Elizabeth O'Brien
Taka Oguisso
Geraldine Padilla
Maria Phaneuf
Jung-Ho Park
Rosemarie Parse
Shannon Perry
Evelyn Peterson
Maria Petursdottir
Maria Phaneuf
Robert Piemonte
Yvonne Pilgrim
Tim Porter-O'Grady
Muriel Poulin
Bhanu Jonathan Ragho
Margaret Reynolds
Rebecca Rimel
Marlene Rosenkoetter
Brenda Roberts
Bonny Roche
Judith Ryan
Marla Salmon
Dolores Sands

Sarah Sanford
Kathleen Scharer
Jacklon Schmidt
Doris Schwartz
Jozefína Sepe iová
Sherry Shamansky
Iris Shannon
Lilly Shortridge
Lillian Simms
Dorothy Smith
Shirley Smoyak
S. Srilatha
Kirsten Stallknecht
Regina Stefnisdottir
Phyllis Stern
Lisa Stevens
Jane Stilwell-Smith
Neville Strumpf
Gail Stuart
Dorothy Talbot
Susan Talbott
Robert Tiffany
    (deceased)
Elizabeth Tornquist
Mary Jane Trautman
Florence Trout
Sallie Tucker-Allen
Suzanne Van Ort
Donna Ver Steeg
Linda Walsh
Mabel Wandelt
Verle Waters
Jean Watson
Fay Whitney
Carolyn Williams
Gay Williams
Holly Wilson
Beatrice Crofts Yorker

Angelou, M. From the book *I Dream a World: Portraits of Black Women Who Changed America,* copyright © 1989, Brian Lanker. Reprinted by permission of Stewart, Tabori & Chang, Publishers, New York.

Anonymous. "Hello David, My Name is Dusty." From CALIFORNIA NURSING REVIEW. Excerpted and adapted with permission of the publisher.

Anzaldúa, G. "Foreword: What to Do from Here and How?" in THIS BRIDGE CALLED MY BACK. Copyright © 1983 by Cherríe Moraga and Gloria Anzaldúa. Used by permission of the author and of Kitchen Table: Women of Color Press, P.O. Box 908, Latham, N.Y. 12110.

Aptheker, B. Excerpts reprinted from TAPESTRIES OF LIFE: WOMEN'S WORK, WOMEN'S CONSCIOUSNESS, AND THE MEANING OF DAILY EXPERIENCE by Bettina Aptheker (Amherst: University of Massachusetts Press, 1989), copyright © 1989 by the University of Massachusetts Press.

Bateson, M. C. Excerpts from the book COMPOSING A LIFE, copyright © 1989 by Catherine Bateson. Used with the permission of the Atlantic Monthly Press.

Beethoven, L. V. Heiligenstadt testament. Reprinted from THE LETTERS OF BEETHOVEN edited by Emily Anderson, by permission of W.W. Norton & Company Inc. Copyright © 1966 by W.W. Norton & Company, Inc.

Bellah, R., Madsen, R., Sullivan, W. M., Swiddler, A., & Tipton, S. M. (1985). Excerpts from HABITS OF THE HEART: INDIVIDUALISM AND COMMITMENT IN AMERICAN LIFE. Copyright © 1985 The Regents of the University of California.

Bird, R. "A Daughter's Story" by Rose Bird. From STANFORD NURSE, Winter, 1992. Reprinted with permission of Stanford Nurse.

Buchanan, J. H. "The Face of the Wolf." From PATIENT ENCOUNTERS: THE EXPERIENCE OF DISEASE, by James H. Buchanan (Charlottesville: Virginia, 1989). Reprinted by permission of the University Press of Virginia.

Callahan, D. "The Priority of Care over Cure." From WHAT KIND OF LIFE. Copyright © 1990 by Daniel Callahan. Reprinted by permission of Simon & Schuster, Inc.

Carter, L. "Only Human" by Lu Carter. From the WESTERN JOURNAL OF MEDICINE, July, 1991, p. 82. with permission of the author.

Casteñada, L. Cashier and Line Stocker. Taken from *Women and Work: Photographs and Personal Writings,* by Maureen R. Michelson, New Sage Press, 1986. Reprinted by permission.

Christ, C. Excerpt from DIVING DEEP AND SURFACING by Carol P. Christ. Copyright © 1980 by Carol P. Christ. Reprinted by permission of Beacon Press.

Collins, B. T. (1988, November/December). "Letter to the Editor." From CALIFORNIA NURSING REVIEW. Excerpted and adapted with permission of the publisher.

Collins, J. Midwives. Taken from *Women and Work: Photographs and Personal Writings,* by Maureen R. Michelson, New Sage Press, 1986. Reprinted by permission.

Cousins, N. Reprinted from ANATOMY OF AN ILLNESS, As Perceived by the Patient, by Norman Cousins, by permission of W.W. Norton & Company, Inc. Copyright © 1979 by W.W. Norton & Company, Inc.

Cousins, N. Reprinted from THE HEALING HEART: Antidotes to Panic and Helplessness, by Norman Cousins, by permission of W.W. Norton & Company, Inc. Copyright © 1983 by Norman Cousins.

Cowan, J. Excerpts from SMALL DECENCIES: REFLECTIONS AND MEDITATIONS ON BEING HUMAN AT WORK by John Cowan. Copyright © 1992 by John Cowan. Reprinted by permission of HarperCollins Publishers Inc.

Curtin, L. "Maria's Choice" by Leah Curtin. From NURSING MANAGEMENT, Vol. 21, No. 11, pages 7–8. Permission requested from and granted by Nursing Management.

Dass, R., & Gorman, P. Excerpts from HOW CAN I HELP? by Ram Dass and Paul Gorman. Copyright © 1985 by Ram Dass and Paul Gorman. Reprinted by permission of Alfred A Knopf, Inc.

de Beauvoir, S. Excerpts from A VERY EASY DEATH by Simone deBeauvoir, translated by Patrick O'Brien. Translation copyright © 1965 by Andre Deutsch Ltd., George Weidenfeld and Nicolson Ltd., and G. P. Putnam's Sons. Reprinted by permission of Pantheon Books, a division of Random House, Inc.

Dickinson, E. "There's Been a Death" and "Hope is a Thing with Feathers." Reprinted by permission of the publishers and the Trustees of Amherst College from THE POEMS OF EMILY DICKINSON, Thomas H. Johnson, ed., Cambridge, Mass.: The Belknap Press of Harvard University Press, Copyright © 1951, 1955, 1979, 1983 by the President and Fellows of Harvard College.

Dickinson, E. The mystery of pain. COLLECTED POEMS OF EMILY DICKINSON. New York: Avenel Books (c/o Outlet Book Company). Reprinted with permission of Little, Brown and Company and Harvard University Press.

Diers, D. "Learning: The Art and Craft of Nursing" by Donna Diers. Copyright © 1991 The American Journal of Nursing Company. Reprinted from the AMERICAN JOURNAL OF NURSING, January 1991, Vol. 91, No. 1. Used with permission. All rights reserved.

Eliot, T. S. "The Love Song of J. Alfred Prufrock" from COLLECTED POEMS 1909–1962 by T. S. Eliot, copyright © 1936 by Harcourt Brace & Company, copyright © 1964, 1963 by T. S. Eliot, reprinted by permission of the publisher.

Estes, C. P. From WOMEN WHO RUN WITH THE WOLVES by Clarissa Pinkola Estes. Copyright © 1992 by Clarissa Pinkola Estes. Reprinted by permission of Ballantine Books, a division of Random House, Inc.

Fagin, C., & Diers, D. "Nursing as Metaphor," by Claire Fagin and Donna Diers. From the NEW ENGLAND JOURNAL OF MEDICINE, July 14, 1983, Vol. 309, pages 116–117. Reprinted with permission from the New England Journal of Medicine.

Fishbein, J. "The Poetry of Medicine" by J. Fishbein. JOURNAL OF THE AMERICAN MEDICAL ASSOCIATION, 264(23), 2999. Copyright © 1988/90, American Medical Association.

Frank, A. W. Excerpts from AT THE WILL OF THE BODY by Arthur Frank. Copyright © 1991 by Arthur Frank. Reprinted by permission of Houghton Mifflin Company. All rights reserved.

Frost, R. "Education by Poetry: A Meditative Monologue from SELECTED PROSE OF ROBERT FROST edited by Hyde Cox and Edward Connery Lathem. Copyright © 1966 by Henry Holt and Company, Inc.

Frost, R. "The Road Not Taken. From THE POETRY OF ROBERT FROST edited by Edward Connery Lathem. Copyright © 1916, 1969 by Henry Holt and Company, Inc. Copyright © 1944 by Robert Frost. Reprinted by permission of Henry Holt and Company, Inc.

Gordon, S. "What Nurses Know" by Suzanne Gordon in MOTHER JONES, September–October, 1992, pp. 41–46. Reprinted with permission of the author and publisher.

Gordon, S. From PRISONERS OF MEN'S DREAMS: STRIKING OUT FOR A NEW FEMININE FUTURE by Suzanne Gordon. Copyright © 1991 by Suzanne Gordon. By permission of Little, Brown and Company.

Hall, S. "Gail." IN HEALTH, pp. 62–69. Reprinted from IN HEALTH, Copyright © 1990.

Hammarskjöld, D. From MARKINGS by Dag Hammarskjöld, translated by Leif Sjöberg & W. H. Auden. Translation copyright © 1984 by Alfred A. Knopf and Faber & Faber Ltd. Reprinted by permission of Alfred A. Knopf, Inc.

Havel, V. Excerpt from LETTERS TO OLGA by V. Havel. Copyright © 1989, by V. Havel. Reprinted by permission of Alfred A. Knopf, Inc.

Hedgeman, A. A. From the book *I Dream a World: Portraits of Black Women Who Changed America,* copyright © 1989, Brian Lanker. Reprinted by permission of Stewart, Tabori & Chang, Publishers, New York.

Joseph, J. "Warning" by Jenny Joseph. In S. Martz (Ed.), WHEN I AM AN OLD WOMAN I SHALL WEAR PURPLE. Watsonville, CA: Papier Mache Press. Copyright John Johnson, Ltd., London.

King, M. L. "I Have A Dream." Reprinted by arrangement with the Heirs of the Estate of Martin Luther King Jr., c/o Joan Daves Agency as agent for the proprietor. Copyright © 1963 by Martin Luther King, Jr., copyright renewed 1991 by Coretta Scott King.

Koller, A. Working, from THE STATIONS OF SOLITUDE by Alice Koller, William Morrow & Company. Copyright © 1990 by Alice Koller. Reprinted by permission of the author.

Lenburg, C. "Out of the Hard Places" by Carrie Lenburg. In T. Schorr & A. Zimmerman (Eds.), MAKING CHOICES, TAKING CHANCES: NURSE LEADERS TELL THEIR STORIES. Reprinted with permission from Mosby-Year Book, Inc.

Lerner, M. Reprinted from WRESTLING WITH THE ANGEL: A Memoir of My Triumph over Illness by Max Lerner, by permission of W.W. Norton & Company, Inc. Copyright © 1990 by Max Lerner.

Lester, C. "Carmelita Lester." From WORKING by Studs Terkel. Copyright © 1972, 1974 by Studs Terkel. Reprinted by permission of Pantheon Books, a division of Random House, Inc.

LeSueur, M. "Rites of Ancient Ripening" copyright © 1982 by Meridel LeSueur. Reprinted from *Ripening: Selected works, 1927–1980.* Published by The Feminist Press at The City University of New York.

Levine, S. "The Healing for Which We Took Birth." Reprinted by permission of The Putnam Publishing Group from HEALERS ON HEALING by Richard Carlson, Ph.D. and Benjamin Shield. Copyright © 1989 by Richard Carlson and Benjamin Shield.

Lindbergh, A. M. "Broken Shell" and "Family Album" from THE UNICORN AND OTHER POEMS: 1935–1955 by Anne Morrow Lindbergh. Copyright © 1956 by Anne Morrow Lindbergh and renewed 1984 by Anne Morrow Lindbergh. Reprinted by permission of Pantheon Books, a division of Random House, Inc.

Linfield, D. "How do I tell my daughter?" THE NEW YORK TIMES, June 3, 1992. Copyright © 1992 by The New York Times Company. Reprinted by permission.

Livingston, G. "Dear Lucas" by G. Livingston. In the SAN FRANCISCO CHRONICLE, *Image Magazine,* November 8, pp. 28–29. Reprinted with permission of the author.

Mallison, M. "How Can You Bear To Be A Nurse?" by Mary Mallison. Copyright © 1987 The American Journal of Nursing Company. Reprinted from the AMERICAN JOURNAL OF NURSING, April, 1987, Vol. 87, No. 5. Used with permission. All rights reserved.

Masson, V. "The Art of the Matter" by Veneta Masson. Reproduced from NURSING OUTLOOK, Vol. 39, No. 4, page 187 with permission from Mosby-Year Book, Inc.

Millay, E. S. V. "To the Wife of a Sick Friend," by Edna St. Vincent Millay. From COLLECTED POEMS, HarperCollins. Copyright © 1928, 1955, by Edna St. Vincent Millay and Norma Millay Ellis. Reprinted by permission of Elizabeth Barnett, Literary executor.

Millay, E. S. V. "Lament," by Edna St. Vincent Millay. From COLLECTED POEMS, HarperCollins. Copyright © 1921, 1948, by Edna St. Vincent Millay. Reprinted by permission of Elizabeth Barnett, Literary executor.

Miller, E. E. "Trust and Honesty: Foundations of Healing." Reprinted by permission of The Putnam Publishing Group from HEALERS ON HEALING by Richard

Author Index

SUBJECT INDEX